ATTACHMENT AND EARLY HOSPITALIZATION

ATTACHMENT AND EARLY HOSPITALIZATION

AN EXPERIMENT IN THE PREVENTION OF
POSTHOSPITAL DISTURBANCE IN INFANTS

JOOP FAHRENFORT

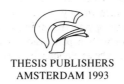

THESIS PUBLISHERS
AMSTERDAM 1993

CIP-DATA KONINKLIJKE BIBLIOTHEEK, DEN HAAG

Fahrenfort, Joop

Attachment and early hospitalization : an experiment in
the prevention of posthospital disturbance in infants /
Joop Fahrenfort. - Amsterdam : Thesis Publishers
Also publ. as thesis Leiden, 1993. - With ref. - With
summary in Dutch.
ISBN 90-5170-215-9
NUGI 712/741
Subject headings: infants ; hospitals ; attachment

Foto's omslag: Inge Baauw
Omslagontwerp: Mirjam Bode

ISBN 90-5170-215-9
NUGI 712/741

CONTENTS

INTRODUCTION

The idea of research into disturbances of infants which may be brought about by hospitalization originated during theoretical explorations in the Department of Phoniatrics of Utrecht University some years before the project was actually initiated. The psychobiological theme at the time was the effect of stressful experience on early development. The hypothesis to be articulated suggested that minor stress could be beneficial in emotional development, whereas excessive stress for infants could be a cause of disturbance as well as an impediment to recovery from somatic illness. A well known example of stressful experience is the separation of infants from their caregivers, which has for many years been a central concern of attachment theory. Attachment theory explains the *degree of distress* that some *infants* in hospital are liable to when parents are absent, even for a limited stretch of time. The initial hypothesis, by interpreting possible traumatic effects of hospitalization as effects of excessive stress, predicted harmful consequences for development. The literature on hospitalization in childhood confirmed that such effects had sometimes been found, for instance in Douglas' influential but now outdated study, that will be discussed in our first chapter. The empirical knowledge of short-term effects of hospitalization, frequently called *upset*, is considerable. On the other hand the possible long-term effects have not been studied sufficiently.

Impressions of current practice suggested that the *specific hazards for infants* might still be underestimated, although attention to the needs of children in general had become a popular concern. For example, much attention is being paid to the general "child-orientedness" of a hospital, which may be evident in a number of provisions and rules. On the vital issue of rooming-in the common policy at present is that it should be possible, but the fact that some parents choose to do it, while others do not, is outside the usual scope of hospital policy. This state of affairs fostered the hope that (additional) prevention was possible. The impetus for the present research project was thus derived from theoretical ideas, but also motivated by the hope of prevention. The scarcity of recent research within the relevant age-group reinforced the position that such a project would be useful.

The opportunity to arrange and design a research project on the psychological risks of hospitalization for infants and toddlers under three years of age was found in Leiden University. An application to the *Praeventiefonds* was supported by experts from the field of pediatrics and the domain of attachment theory. Ultimately, of course, these different disciplines do not serve a different cause. The development of plans and designs for research was a shared interdisciplinary enterprise. Finally, the *Fonds* upheld the project. Although execution of the plans had become feasible, many practical problems, that will not be discussed now, were in store for the research team. No less than eight hospitals in six different towns and cities have contributed to (parts of) this research, which required several years for the collection of data.

From the start the theme of the inquiry has been the subsequent adjustment of children who had been hospitalized repeatedly and/or for longer than a few days only, before the age of three years. Chronically hospitalized infants and hospitalized newborn infants were not included, because they suffer from comparatively specific problems. The population studied is larger than these two categories, but smaller than the full population of young children receiving hospital treatment. In the prospective research, which is the *pièce de résistance* of the project, the focus is on surgical patients. The earlier retrospective study suggested this category to be most severely affected. The problems that motivated the project were not the symptoms of short-term upset, which are sometimes recognized without provoking alarm, but suspected long-term symptoms of maladjustment and/or delayed language development. The average term for follow-up after discharge was three years in the retrospective study and one year in the prospective study.

The project had several goals: assessing the incidence of detrimental effects and the duration of symptoms, identifying influential conditions, particularly aspects of parental support and, last but not least, evaluating by experimental design the effects of counseling parents in order to improve, if possible, their participation during treatment of their infant.

The prospective study can be compared to the many research projects into the sequelae of hospitalization that are discussed in the first chapter. The design is distinctive in several ways. In prior investigations the period available for follow-up was usually six months or less. Typically the sample was restricted to minor surgery like tonsillectomy and to one hospital setting. The research to be presented has none of these restrictions. Moreover: for the first time parental support is decomposed into the dimensions of sensitivity and presence in hospital.

The exposition can be subdivided in the following way:
- one chapter is devoted to three subjects, important in their own right: past research, hospital policy and theory;
- one chapter is a complete account of the retrospective study;
- four chapters contain the plan and the outcomes of the larger prospective study;
- one chapter, the final one, contains the critical discussion of the prospective study, the theoretical interpretation of all findings and recommendations for hospital policy.

The parts distinguished can be read separately. Even the interpretations and recommendations in the final part can be understood, given a few references, without full knowledge of the preceding chapters. A detailed summary in Dutch is provided. The four parts will now be introduced one by one.

First part: Past research, hospital policy and theoretical perspectives

These three subjects are treated in the first chapter. First the history of the problem is touched upon: the medical approach of fifty to sixty years ago, which was not much concerned with emotional ties. The early research is arranged, following the book of Vernon and his co-workers in 1965. The non-medical risk of hospitalization was acknowledged then, posthospital disturbance was explained by a number of factors, one of which was the intermittent separation from parents. Subsequent (i.e. after 1965) research of the hypothesis that rooming-in reduces posthospital disturbance is summarized. Most attention is devoted to studies suggesting that posthospital disturbance may influence development of the patient for a number of years.

The evolution which took place between the sixties and the nineties has thoroughly changed hospital practices and traditions, at least in western Europe and the U.S.A. This is described in the second section. Anno 1990 rooming-in is usually allowed and sometimes stimulated. It is not, however, for children at risk a universal precaution.

The third section presents theory and research. The vulnerability of young children to separations is explained by the basic tenets of attachment theory. The framework is extended with experiments in substitute care, neurophysiological assessments of stress and research pertaining to attachment quality. Three categories of attachment relationships are commonly distinguished by the current research tradition. Secure attachment may be a protective factor. On the other hand secure attachment may give way to avoidant attachment, because of separation or other stress in hospital. Parental support is thus presumed to be of vital influence. It is divided into presence (implying involvement) during the various episodes of the hospital treatment, and sensitivity of the parent during video-recorded interactions with the child.

Second part: The retrospective study

The retrospective study, which is described in the second chapter, was designed to compare the current behavior problems of a sample of former patients, selected for their hospitalization history, with a non-hospitalized control group. The specific advantage of the retrospective design is the possibility to select a sample of children with various degrees of hospitalization experience. Effects of hospitalization on behavior several years after the latest discharge were investigated. An increase of problem behavior was detected. Effects of parental presence in hospital (as remembered and reported by the parent later on) were not as clear cut as had been expected; other factors were identified as predictive in exploratory analysis. The outcomes are discussed in Section 2.5.

Third part: The prospective study

A formal description of the method of this study is given in Chapter 3, after a succinct statement of the purpose and of the eleven hypotheses, mainly derived from the theory and literature in the first chapter. The figures 3.1 and 3.2 contain this information in a highly condensed form. The design includes visits to the family before admission, during admission, and several times after discharge. Constructs are quantified with the help of questionnaires, interviews, standardized tests and coding of videotaped child-parent interactions. By design an experimental group (receiving interventions to stimulate parental support) and a control group have been are distinguished.

Chapter 4 contains the technical works. First the sample of 64 cases is described, as regards medical history and various conventional characteristics. Meanwhile the design-groups are compared in terms of independent variables; minor flaws are detected. Next the instruments are reviewed psychometrically. The following variables have eventually been constructed, measured and prepared for the testing of hypotheses.
antecedent conditions:
- hospitalization history
- preadmission adjustment / behavior problems
dynamics of interaction:
- parental sensitivity
- initial attachment security
- parental attendance in hospital
post-test / follow-up criteria:
- short-term upset after discharge
- behavior problems (maladjustment) during follow-up
- disturbance of relationship to caregiver
- ego-resilience
- language development
An overview of the interrelations among these objects of thought is presented in Chapter 5, Figure 5.1. This is relevant to the procedure of testing hypotheses. Next the method of analysis, analysis of covariance, is described. The results of hypothesis testing comprise the rest of the chapter. Effects of interventions are treated in Section 5.4 and quasi-experimental effects of parental support in Section 5.5. Some important data are not included in Chapter 5, because they are not involved in hypothesis testing. These are saved for Chapter 6, a short chapter. It contains three unrelated subjects: the value of rooming-in, the characteristic developmental problems of children in different medical categories, and the decline of adjustment in the sample. The

methodological problems of the prospective study are reviewed in terms of validity, in Section 7.1.

Fourth part: Final results (Chapter 7)

For many readers the most interesting part will be the empirical conclusions and their theoretical interpretations. First the technical aspects of the theoretical interpretation are discussed as validity issues in Section 7.1. The final conclusion for each hypothesis is summarized in Section 7.2. A deeper theoretical statement in terms of presumed underlying processes, is presented in Section 7.3. This section, of course, takes the findings of prior research into consideration. It includes comment on the possible interplay of cognitive and emotional/relational processes, a difficult subject for this age-category, worthy of additional research.

The most palpable results are recommendations, formulated in the last section of the book. These represent a modest program, based on previous findings as well as on newly acquired knowledge. The heart of the matter seems to be the recognition and acknowledgement of non-medical risk.

CHAPTER 1   EMOTIONAL IMPACT OF HOSPITALIZATION

The aim of this chapter is to sketch the subject matter: a problem, that became a field of research halfway through our century. Section 1.1 gives an outline of this history and a description of lines of research. Specific attention is given to studies that consider long-term sequelae of hospitalization and the value of rooming-in. In Section 1.2 an account is given of past and present hospital policy concerning parental participation. Section 1.3 offers a description of theoretical viewpoints that have influenced the present study. One viewpoint is biological and ethological research in which the concepts of stress and coping are linked to neuroendocrine assessments. A second viewpoint, which has been more influential in the research design adopted later, is the attachment theory of, among others, John Bowlby and Mary Ainsworth.

1.1   Research on hospitalized children in historical perspective

Early viewpoints

Interest in the psychological effects of hospital experiences in childhood is largely a phenomenon of the last fifty years. The earliest communication on this subject identified in our search is that of Beverly (1936) who recognized the emotional troubles of infants and children during and after hospitalization. He was the first to appoint a "play lady", many years before such an official was commonly found to be useful. He even made a hesitant proposal that children should be visited daily by their parents.

It seems likely that the policy and practice of hospital care sixty years ago have produced victims never recognized as such. This is illustrated by the work of Stades Veth (1973, 1981). Between 1930 and 1940 she conducted play therapy with toddlers referred for psychiatric treatment in Leiden. In 1970, upon a renewed analysis of material from this period and additional data, she decided that hospital experiences had been the principal cause of the severe disturbances of these children. Afterwards, still very early within the Dutch perspective, she wrote ardently on the dangers of early hospitalization. At the time of treatment neither parents nor she herself as therapist made this attribution.

It should be remembered that theories concerning infant-caregiver attachment, including older concepts like "maternal deprivation" were developed rather late in this century. As related in a historical sketch by Hunt (1974) a child in hospital was formerly considered to be a biological unit, not a part of a (family-) system. This is vividly documented in the pioneering study of Edelston (1943). He describes 44 cases of children, whose severe disturbances can be related, by case-history, to hospital admissions, which were sometimes prolonged for months, often without parental visiting. As to the issue of visiting Edelston quotes an editorial in the Lancet:

> *The child does not need visitors in the same way as does the adult patient and*
> *this means any visiting (...) is for the benefit of the parents rather than the*

patients. If this is accepted it is surely logical to forbid visiting altogether. (Jan. 27, 1940)
Edelston:
This statement called forth but one single criticism besides my own. Dr. J.M. Bowlby wrote protesting against this cavalier dismissal of the psychological side of the problem.

The usual practice at the time was to allow "a limited number of visits, provided (!) the child is not unduly disturbed" by them. At least as important as this historical issue is the theoretical explanation provided by Edelston of the sometimes traumatizing effects of hospitalization. The later attachment-theory as expounded by Bowlby is present here in embryonic form:

I should like to suggest that where the child's appeal (open or implied) for assistance and comfort is not answered by the parent the enhanced feelings of distress aroused are identical with the anxiety resulting from "loss of the mother" as previously described; or to use another terminology, with the emotional insecurity following rejection. (...)
Observation of young infants shows that the infant recognizes the face of the mother (or nurse) at an earlier age than it recognizes the bottle; its gestures are directed towards the person and not towards the object of gratification.

The earliest systematic research on the subject of childhood hospitalization was conducted in the early fifties. Jackson, Winkley, Faust, Cermak and Burtt (1952) came up against many methodological complexities in this "new type of research". A better example is the study of Prugh, Staub, Sands, Kirschbaum and Lenihan (1953). In addition to statistical comparisons careful descriptions and interpretations are given in their substantial report, concerning a hundred children, aged 2-12. Of course methodological standards in those days were less strict than today. It is not germane to give a full description of this research; however, one conclusion may be quoted.

Children under four years of age and children who had unsatisfying relationships with their parents, who had undergone very severe stress in the hospital and who had shown the greatest difficulty in adapting to the ward milieu were those who tended to show persistent signs of emotional disturbance at three months following hospitalization.

The citation list of Prugh et al. (1953) testified to the spreading awareness of the research-field discussed here, and of the importance of the problems in question. At about the same time Robertson produced, in Britain, his film document on the hospitalization of a two year old girl (Robertson, 1952). In the work of Bowlby (1953) the concept of maternal deprivation was paramount.

In 1965 a fully comprehensive and careful review of the already voluminous literature on psychological responses of children to hospitalization and illness was prepared and published by Vernon, Foley, Sipowicz and Schulman. It is useful to summarize their conclusions here:
(1)   There is, according to Vernon and co-workers, no serious doubt about the risk of psychological upset associated with hospitalization. Among studies of changes from prehospital to posthospital periods the most common finding has been that more children change in the direction of upset than change in the direction of benefit. These findings are compatible with the evidence of a few studies where nonhospital control groups are

16

employed. Nevertheless many children may experience hospitalization and emerge unharmed, or even improved.

(2)   Whilst the earliest explanations of adverse response are related to the separation between child-patient and parents (in the past usually represented by the mother), a number of determinants may contribute to the observed effects. Vernon et al. (1965) discuss the unfamiliarity of the hospital setting, sensory-motor restrictions, age, prehospital personality and some other possible determinants. They do *not* consider these to be *competing* hypotheses.

(3)   The proposal that unfamiliarity could be a source of disturbance received considerable support from investigations of psychological preparation. Preparing the child tends to decrease the incidence of psychological upset.

(4)   Data relevant to the effects of separation indicated that it contributes to upset, both during and immediately following hospitalization; however, according to Vernon: "it is unlikely" that this factor entails long-term consequences for emotional adjustment.

(5)   Investigations concerning age suggested a curvilinear relationship between this variable and psychological upset. Children between approximately six months and three to four years appeared to be particularly vulnerable.

(6)   Data concerning prehospital personality provided limited support for the hypothesis that poor prior adjustment is likely to be associated with more frequent or more severe upset.

(7)   Changes were apparent (in 1965) in terms of liberal visiting policies, programs to prepare children for surgery, play rooms and more liberal rules concerning bed-rest. One would anticipate that hospitalization, when accompanied by these ameliorating circumstances, would be less traumatic than the literature indicates.

Many of the cautiously worded conclusions of Vernon et al. (1965) have been reaffirmed in later research, the cumulative changes, indicated in statement 7, notwithstanding. Several of these propositions, like (3) and (5), remain firm, others need a replication for the present (1990) situation. Long term follow-up in particular was scant at the time of this review. The statement that effects of separation are not likely to have long-term consequences, apparently based on two retrospective studies (Stott, 1956; Howells & Layng, 1955) seems ill founded, when compared to other results.

Directions of research after 1965

The years after 1965 have witnessed an impressive growth in the literature on pediatric hospitalization. The lines of research discussed by Vernon et al. (1965) have been expanded. From our viewpoint the most significant widening of scope has been the appearance of longitudinal research concerning long-term sequelae of hospitalization. This subject will be covered in the next few sections. It is a curious fact that on this critical issue our knowledge is clearly insufficient (Yap, 1988a; Fahrenfort, 1989).

The effect of parental presence on posthospital maladjustment has received due attention. Since restrictions on visiting have been abandoned the practice of rooming-in has been the focus of attention in this respect. Findings will be reviewed at the end of this section (p. 21).

The subject that has drawn most attention is psychological preparation. As a rule such preparation is found to be advantageous for children of four years and older (Thompson, 1985). For younger children preparatory programs are not considered feasible. In one major study Wolfer and Visintainer (1979) compared the effectiveness of five conditions: stress-point preparation, home-booklet preparation, a combination of these two, home preparation plus supportive care and a control condition. Each of the experimental conditions resulted in lower levels of children's upset, as well as greater parent satisfaction, but no significant differences between them were obtained. In a few studies it was found that presentation of filmed material preceding surgery for children in the age range 4-17 years may increase anxiety for some subjects. This sensitizing effect was found for younger children scheduled for surgery on the same day who had prior surgical experience (Melamed, Dearborn & Hermecz, 1983; Faust & Melamed, 1984). In a meta-analysis of 75 controlled intervention studies Saile, Burgmeier and Schmidt (1988) found a general mean effect size of half a standard deviation. The effect was larger in the case of severe operations and when the child's well-being was seriously threatened. Surveys of preparation practices in the U.S.A. indicate that practice lags behind the knowledge in this field (Thompson, 1985). Still 74% of pediatric hospitals reported in 1980 that some formal preparation was offered to some patients. An extensive review of findings on efficacy of preparation is provided by Yap (1988b).

Children's conceptions of illness have been addressed by a number of researchers. Like the subject of preparation this topic is age-restricted. The available research concerns children aged four years and older. Studies prior to 1965 repeatedly documented a common childhood belief that illness is the product of one's own action and accordingly treatment may be viewed as punishment. Of nine *subsequent* studies examining hospitalized and/or nonhospitalized subjects' conceptions of illness, six confirmed that children, especially young children, consider illness to be self-caused and are apt to view the resulting conditions as punishment. (Thompson, 1985). This view is especially prevalent among young, chronically ill children and tends to decline with age. Although the meaning of this piece of knowledge for even younger children is not certain, the possible relevance of immature cognitions should be borne in mind.

Manifestations of upset or maladjustment

Throughout the review of Vernon et al., as well as in the more recent comprehensive review of Thompson (1985) a distinction is made between *immediate responses*, in the sense of behavior observed in hospital, and *posthospital responses*, observed after discharge. In Thompson (1985) the category of *long-term responses*, in the sense of behavior one or more years after discharge, has been added.

Behavior during hospitalization, the *immediate response*, has been studied to obtain measures of distress or upset exhibited under different conditions. Unlike posthospital response the relevance or meaning of any immediate response may be disputed. As it is not relevant at present, measures of immediate response will not be discussed.

Posthospital behavior is the most revealing manifestation of possible adverse effects of hospitalization. The nature of behavioral disturbances in the first few months after discharge is listed in many sources, like the major reviews just cited and many original studies (Schaffer & Callender, 1959; Vernon, Schulman & Foley, 1966; Brain & Maclay, 1968; Dearden, 1970; Douglas, 1975; Stades Veth, 1981; Mrazek, 1984). The interpretation of posthospital behavior indicating temporary upset after discharge is facilitated when insecurity, anger, or both are manifest. A typical response of toddlers is clinging to the caregiver and protesting very short separations, even the closing of the door when she needs to use the toilet. At the same time strangers and sometimes even family members like grandparents, are viewed with suspicion or alarm. Resistance at bedtime suggests reluctance to allow separation. Very common are sleep disturbances. Some children wake up every other hour, presumably to check the presence of parents. When reassured they may soon go back to sleep, but never for long. In severe cases children may cry and fail to be comforted, even by the mother. As a last resort parents sometimes decide to take the child in their own bed, even despite their conviction that this is bad policy. In some children behavior becomes more aggressive. The mildest form of aggression is a selfish or uncompromising attitude towards siblings. Typically newborn siblings are rejected and sometimes molested. Aggression towards attachment figures may be expressed in noncompliance, fits, or temper tantrums. Other complaints are eating problems and loss of attainments in toilet training.

This bird's eye view of problematic posthospital behavior can not be exhaustive, and fails to specify individual variety, but may indicate the emotional roots of symptoms, present in some children and absent in others. The prevalence is much higher during the first days or weeks after discharge from hospital than later on. As to the duration of problems, the issue is not whether specific behavior patterns will persist for one or more years, but whether unfavorable dispositions, like fearfulness have been acquired.

When traces of traumatic experience can be established years after hospitalization, the phrase "long-term response" is not very apt. This seems to denote some specific behavior in response to some specific stimulus. Where the connection is established, it is more appropriate to speak of "developmental disturbance" in response to hospitalization. Any observation or measurement considered important by the investigator can be studied as a possible symptom of developmental disturbance. In the research, to be described shortly, ratings of socio-emotional behavior, obtained from parents and teachers, and scores of educational attainment, are employed. In our own study various standardized instruments to measure general adjustment are used. Parental report, mediated by questionnaires, is an important, but by no means the only approach.

Evidence of developmental disturbance

Woodward (1959), in her retrospective study of 198 children hospitalized for severe burns, reported 81% to be slightly, moderately or severely disturbed at the time of follow-up. Emotional disturbance was assessed, two to five years after discharge, on the basis of interviews with the mothers. The corresponding percentage was 7% for 608 siblings of the patients, 14% for a random control group of 50 children, and 12% for 123 siblings of the controls. Of the patients 15% were estimated to be disturbed before the accident. It may be true that these populations were different, but criteria for this comparison are not clearly stated. Woodward's interpretation that much of the disturbance was dependent on lack of parental visiting was consistent with her data, but could not rigorously be demonstrated.

Stott (1959) compared a sample of 142 children, who had been hospitalized under the age of two, for periods of generally two to four weeks, with a control group of normal children similar in age and sex. Reading difficulties, rated by teachers approximately *five to ten years after hospitalization*, were found to be more common among the hospital group (p < .001). Furthermore, reading difficulties were still more frequent among children who had experienced several episodes of illness (p < .01). Stott's analysis and interpretations suggest that the underlying cause might be a general congenital vulnerability in the population studied.

One extensive and careful investigation in this field is that of Douglas (1975). This contribution concerns an eighteen year follow-up of a cohort born in 1946. The main independent variables were frequency and duration of hospital admissions before the age of five years. The main dependent variables were (a) teachers' ratings concerning troublesome behavior outside the class at ages thirteen and fifteen, (b) scores on the Watts-Vernon reading test at age fifteen, (c) delinquent behavior in the 8-17 age range, (d) frequent job changes among those who no longer attended school.

An alarming significant association was found between either repeated or lengthy hospitalization at preschool age and the aforementioned criteria (a) and (b). This association remained significant after successively controlling for (1) readmissions at a later age, (2) persistent physical disabilities, (3) father's occupation, (4) family size, (5) parents' interest in education. The similar relationship between early hospitalization and the criteria (c) and (d) proved to be confounded by later hospitalization. Relationships between precise age of hospitalization under five and follow-up measures, as well as between mothers' reports on behavior after discharge and follow-up measures were consistent with the hypothesis that social and emotional development had been affected by early hospitalization, and that an 8-10 year time span had been insufficient to obliterate the traces of it.

Quinton and Rutter (1976) attempted to replicate the principal findings of Douglas on a sample of nearly four hundred British children. One of their objectives was to consider the possible confounding effects of psychosocial disadvantage in the family. Family adversity might constitute an explanation of both developmental disturbances and a history of early hospital admissions. Their findings indicated that ratings for emotional and conduct disorder at ten years of age were associated with multiple admissions in the first five years, even controlling for psychosocial disadvantage. The statistical effect of lengthy (over one month) single admissions, reported by Douglas, could not be replicated because of limitations of the data. The statistical effect of single admissions in the range of one to four weeks, recorded by Douglas (1975), proved to be absent.

While Quinton and Rutter do not report on hospital policy, Douglas emphasizes that the relevant hospital admissions in his study occurred before 1952, at a time when hospital provisions were far below later standards. In 47% of cases parents were not allowed to visit at all. Only three of the twelve hundred mothers were allowed to stay with their child in hospital.

Insufficient knowledge to judge whether past findings still hold true in the present is a perennial problem in this field. Remarkably little has been done since 1980 to check the situation concerning long-term complaints. The only really relevant study is the latest, also British, cohort study by Haslum (1988). Once again she found some associations between hospitalization experience in the 0-5 age range, and educational attainments as well as behavioral ratings. Children who had been hospitalized for three weeks or more in their preschool years were performing avaragely 0.2 standard deviation below their peers, who had been hospitalized for less than one week. The difference applied to both reading and mathematics test scores at age ten. More revealing as a manifestation of socio-emotional upheaval are ratings by mothers concerning *antisocial* behavior at age five, which proved to be significantly related to multiple admissions in the preceding years. This association remained after linear adjustments for sex of the child, birthweight, parental situation, maternal smoking and number of children in the household. Similarly *inattentive behavior* at age ten was related to occurrence and frequency of admissions, both in the developmental stage before, and after the age of five. Whilst educational delays in hospitalized children, related to length of hospitalization, may not indicate emotional trauma, inattentive or antisocial behavior does. While recently hospitalized children were included in the population studied here, presumably for the majority the observations represented long-term sequelae. Thus available evidence, limited as it appears, is consistent with the hypothesis that, even after 1980, the emotional experience of hospitalization entails long-term disturbance.

Rooming-in

The relevance of rooming-in with the child, to be available as a parent for support and reassurance at night does not require an elaborate discussion. Research on the efficacy of this practice, is summarized in Table 1.1. It appears that in five studies, conducted in Britain, the U.S.A. and Germany the hypothesis that posthospital behavioral problems could be reduced by rooming-in was confirmed (+ signs). In two other studies only a tendency was found in the expected direction (- signs). Saile (1987) found an interaction effect of rooming-in and age, indicating that only children aged between 12-30 months reaped measurable benefits. The beneficial effect of rooming-in within the age-range 1-3 years is consistently confirmed. For practical and ethical reasons experimental and control groups are self-selected in most of these

TABLE 1.1   *Effects of rooming-in judged by reduction of posthospital upset*

+	significant reduction of upset
+/-	significant interactional effect; main effect not significant, still some support was obtained for the hypothesis
-	no significant effect, only a trend

Author	Year	Country	Age	N	Follow-up	Findings
Fagin	1966	USA	0,5-3 yrs	60	1 month	+
Brain & Maclay	1968	UK	2-6 yrs	197	6 months	+
Lehman	1975	USA	3-5 yrs	48	2 weeks	-
Couture	1976	USA	3-6 yrs	31	1 month	-
McGillicuddy	1976	USA	14-48 m	90	1 month	+
Wanschura & Löschenkohl	1979	Germany	5-70 m	86	weeks (?)	+
Scholz	1983	Germany	1-3 yrs	48	2 months	+
Saile	1987	Germany	1-4,5 yrs	80	12 days	+/-

research endeavors. This is a methodological drawback, only partially made up for by control techniques in statistical analysis. Of course additional methodological criticism of these studies is possible, but it would not be fair to dismiss these findings with their trend toward consensus in different settings. The study of Brain and Maclay (1968) is a counter-example for much criticism. Here a design is employed with random assignment to experimental and control group,a design, as in statistical analysis. Of course additional methodological criticism of these studies is possible, but it would not be fair to dismiss these findings with their trend toward consensus in different settings. The study of Brain and Maclay (1968) is a counter-example for much criticism. Here a design is employed with random assignment to experimental and control group, a design, as Saile (1987) comments, ethically possible in those days. The satisfactory number of children, the six months follow-up and the attention to postoperative complications related to rooming-in make this study particularly valuable. Both Brain and Maclay (1968) and Lehman (1975) observed a reduction of physical complications during recovery where rooming-in had been practiced.

1.2   Hospitals and hospital policy

Evolution of hospital policy

In the period 1960-1990 the increased attention to the psychological wellbeing of children has gradually brought about a complete change of policy and practice in the hospitals. We can distinguish changes of attitude by professional workers, introduction and institution of new rules, particularly regarding parent-child-contact, introduction of new professional roles and expansion of facilities for children. Of course standards in all these areas are not clearly established, and it should not be assumed that practices are generally similar in different hospitals.

In addition to changes in care there has been a continuous decline of the average length of a hospitalization episode. Minor surgery, for example, that formerly involved admissions of three or four days, is frequently handled nowadays by means of one-day-admissions. This trend may prevent a great deal of distress.

Changes of essential importance for young children have come about after much discussion, and occasional conflicts. Nonetheless these changes have evolved analogously in different countries, cf. Robertson (1970) for Britain, Bierman (1978) for Germany, Robinson & Clarke (1980) for Canada, Oremland & Oremland (1973) and Goldberger (1987) for the U.S.A., Veeneklaas, Gobée en Van der Kloot Meijburg (1972), Schweizer (1978), Kind en Ziekenhuis (1982, 1987) and Van Beek (1988) for the Netherlands.

Associations of parents have played an important part. In the Netherlands the association "Kind en Ziekenhuis" [Children in Hospital] was founded in 1977. The aim is (was) to change childcare practices in hospitals, to inform parents about emotional consequences of hospitalization, to abolish restrictions like insufficient opportunity for visiting and rooming-in and to promote, by all means, the wellbeing of children in hospital. Similar organizations exist in other countries, such as the Association for the Welfare of Children in Hospital in England and the Association for the Care of Children's Health in the U.S.A. Many of the earliest objectives of these organizations have been attained by means of dialogue and gradual changes in attitude and policy.

Parental care in hospitals

From the viewpoint that young children in hospital need their parents some recommendations are rather obvious. Albeit short separations (where the meaning of 'short' depends on the individual) need not be harmful and should not be avoided, the infant or toddler should be accompanied by a parent as much as possible. This applies to the time spent in regular day-time rituals like washing and feeding, but even more strictly at stressful moments, when the patient is examined by a doctor, when injections are mandatory, when blood is taken or medicines administered. Simple measurements, like the taking of temperature can be, and often are, performed by parents. Extensive presence in the daytime is cumbersome for parents but recommended in any ordinary case.

The same applies to rooming-in. A hospital ward is not a place where children sleep all night. Hagemann, quoted in Thompson (1985), documents that sleep disruptions are common. Very few of 34 children studied were able to sleep uninterruptedly through more than half of the sleep period. Intuitively it would seem that the risk of traumatic experience is comparatively large for infants who wake up during the night and are unexpectedly confronted with the absence of attachment figures. This has been confirmed by the research findings summarized in Table 1.1.

Finally, presence of parents is advocated and nowadays frequently practiced during the induction of anaesthesia. A relationship between parental presence, emotional upheaval and posthospital adjustment is suggested by a few studies. Meyer and Muravchick (1977) found better posthospital adjustment by the PHBQ (an instrument described in Section 4.3) when upheaval was avoided by induction of anaesthesia while the subject was asleep. Hannallah and Rosales (1987) found that presence of parents resulted in significant decrease of upset or turbulent children during the pre-induction and induction period. There was no difference, however, in the conduct of children afterwards at home. The presence of parents during induction does not usually create any severe problems (Page & Morgan-Hughes, 1990). Schofield and White (1989) reported that of 141 parents, 10 were "less than helpful" to the anaesthesist, but only one was "disruptive", as she was very distressed.

The three domains of possible parental participation: presence and care at daytime, especially during stressful events, rooming-in and presence at induction have been debated for many years, but not in vain. The change in rules and practice will now be described. In the past the principal issue was: "Are parents allowed to ...?" Allowed to sleep either at their child's bedside or somewhere else in the hospital, to provide routine care, to be present at induction of anaesthesia and so on. In 1977 the association Kind en Ziekenhuis initiated a survey, from which the following data are extracted:
- In 95% of the wards for toddlers, visiting hours were restricted: frequently four hours or less were dedicated to visiting. Usually the age of visitors was restricted as well; siblings were not allowed (contamination!).
- Presence of parents during stressful treatment was usually prohibited. Only one out of four, of the wards surveyed, reported that parental presence was commonly approved.
- For most hospitals rooming-in was still science fiction. Only 10% responded positively to the question whether any accommodation was available for the exclusive purpose of lodging parents.
- Presence of parents during induction of anaesthesia was not yet a subject of dissension, i.e., it was never allowed.
- Ordinary care like feeding or bathing could be provided by parents to some extent. In spite of the restrictions on visiting, three out of four toddler's wards reported this practice to be common. For the remainder apparently, this was all the domain of the nurse.

In 1990 the variety of rules in different hospitals is still a subject of interest, but rules are no longer the major obstacle. The data to follow are extracted from the guidebook "*Welk ziekenhuis kiest u?*" [How to choose a hospital], published by Kind en Ziekenhuis in 1992. "Open visiting hours" apply to 90% of the hospitals, and otherwise visiting restrictions are not severe. Parents are expected to provide some daily care for their own children, at least in the case of infants and toddlers. Rooming-in with toddlers is officially possible in 95% of the hospitals, provided 'boxes' (separate cubicles) are available; otherwise in 83%. For infants these figures are lower: 92% and 72% respectively. Most disagreement concerning hospital rules is currently focussed on the presence of parents during induction of anaesthesia and after surgery, in the recovery room. According to their official statements 60% of the hospitals accept the former and 33% the latter demand in cases of elective surgery for toddlers. But frequently actual practice depends on the motivation (persistence) of parents or on the individual anaesthesist concerned. The reason given for restrictions is usually insufficient (spatial) accommodations, which sometimes may be a true motive, sometimes a formal point. Some anaesthesiologists do not feel comfortable when parents are present.

In the debate about hospital rules the appearance may have been created that parents are always eager to be present and involved. Unfortunately, parents sometimes lack the opportunity, or the endurance, or the motivation to be consistently present. Moreover attitudes on the part of the staff are sometimes more influential than rules: parents may be invited and stimulated to be present or they may be discouraged.

The most recent national data on what parents actually do are published in Kind en Ziekenhuis (1987). These figures, perhaps outdated, suggest that parental participation is not as frequent or adequate as hospital rules theoretically make possible. An impression can be gained from Table 1.2. A problem with Table 1.2 is the fact that not parents, but heads of children's wards are the respondents. So the table should be read as follows: in 37% of wards rooming-in occurs most of the time. The vagueness is in the data. More recent and more detailed data on this subject will be reported for the sample of the prospective investigation in Chapter 4.

TABLE 1.2   *Parental participation or presence as reported by heads of children's wards (Kind en Ziekenhuis, 1987). N = 147. Percentages apply to wards, not to parents*

	always or most of the time	sometimes	rarely or never
presence of parents during aggravating interventions	78%	20%	2%
parents rooming-in at night	37%	50%	14%
parents present at induction of anaesthesia	11%	14%	75%

Care by hospital staff

The emphasis placed here on parent-child contacts as a factor in preventing traumatic experience should not obscure the vital importance of the hospital staff: nurses, play leaders, physicians and sometimes psychologists, pedagogues, teachers or social workers. Elaborate description of the role and contribution of these professionals is not relevant to our research. Teachers and social workers do not participate in the care of infants. Psychologists or pedagogues (with academic degree) are not usually involved in the regular clinical care. Their contribution is limited to cases where support has been sought by parents or, infrequently, when psychological problems of patients have attracted the attention of the medical staff. The role of nurses and pedagogical assistants (play leaders) is for the majority of children more significant.

The atmosphere on children's wards in different hospitals can be vastly different, e.g., on some wards it is possible for crying infants without parents to be left unattended for some time, because of workpressure, whereas on other wards this would be unthinkable. Crowding may be common, or may never happen, and a host of other important conditions may be different.

In some sense nurses are necessarily substitute caretakers, when parents are absent. Therefore experiments in substitute care may be relevant. Robertson and Robertson (1967, 1968a, 1968b) have demonstrated that the nature of substitute care during 'brief' (a number of days) separations may effect an invaluable difference in outcome. They produced filmdocuments on the behavior of toddlers, separated from their family, either in a residential nursery or lodged in the Robertson home, provided with care by Mrs. Robertson. Upon consideration of the differential results, Rutter (1981) concludes, after extensive discussion that continuing intense personal interaction with the same individuals during the separation episode is the crucial factor preventing excessive distress. Recognition of this factor in hospital settings has for some wards resulted in a system where primary responsibility for each child patient is assigned to a specific nurse. This principle is already advocated by Robertson (1970) under the name 'case-assignment'. From the infant's point of view this system of nursing is clearly to be preferred. However, in the care for each child other staff-members will also be involved.

The possibilities for a nurse or other caretaker to offer a substitute for attachment figures should not be overestimated. There is little opportunity to extend interactions in time. Smith (cited in Goldberger, 1987) measured duration of any interaction between child-patient and staff. He found a mean *short of 1,5 minutes per interaction*. Grant (1983, summarized in Thompson, 1985) documented the frequency with which people entered a six-bed unit of a children's hospital in New Zealand. On five separate days the number of people entering the room, their identity, and their length of stay was recorded. During an average day, from 6.00 to 18.00, 327 separate entrances were made by 106 different people. Members of the nursing staff accounted for the greatest number of both entrances and individuals entering the unit, followed by visitors, and then doctors. The majority of "visits" was less than one minute in length. Imagine the experience of this setting from the perspective of the child-patient.

In the literature we have not identified much research on differences of sensitivity as an aspect of nursing care, nor have we found any opportunity to include this aspect in the present study. It is likely that differences between nurses are considerable, as were differences between parents. Presumably sensitive nursing is important to patients and to their parents. One study (Mahaffy, 1965) impressively documents how wellbeing of child-patients can be enhanced by a nurse who focusses on the needs of parents. This study demonstrated the benefits of *experimental nursery*, defined by the researcher as *creating upon admission and carrying forth, throughout the hospitalization, a sincere and warm acquaintance between the parent and nurse, which permitted them to communicate freely with each other*. The nurse attempted to relieve parent's discomfort or any other obstacle hampering their caretaking in the hospital. This rather "soft" approach was judged by its effect on physiological measures related to the recovery of the child. Mean temperature, systolic blood pressure and pulse rates of experimental children proved to be significantly lower than those of controls: preoperatively, postoperatively and at discharge. Total volume and ease of fluid intake following surgery were also greater among children in the experimental group. Incidence of vomiting was lower than in the control group. Parent reports after discharge indicated fewer medical problems and swifter recovery among experimental children.

An important figure for many child-patients is the *pedagogical assistant* or co-worker, in the past usually designated 'play-leader', sometimes 'observer' (Veeneklaas et al., 1972), and at present in the USA 'child life worker'. The qualifications and responsibility of such assistants are not the same in all wards. A basic task of the pedagogical assistant is to provide opportunity for play activities, including supervision and supply of facilities, toys and other materials. This commonly involves sessions in the play-room, at fixed hours in the morning and/or the afternoon. Some children are able to play without any restriction, others are obviously too ill, some can be allowed in the play-room with drip-apparatus or in bed. The assistant may provide individual opportunities for play for children who cannot participate in play sessions; however, such attention is not available for any child that needs it. Apart from tasks related to play-opportunities, the pedagogical assistant frequently has a general responsibility for the wellbeing of the child. This may include preparing the child for surgery, acquainting him/her with attributes such as surgical dressing and supporting parents when they attend the induction of anaesthesia. Obviously, like the nurse, the pedagogical assistant may influence the wellbeing of child-patient and parents during hospitalization. Our study design did not permit evaluation of her actual contribution, which may depend on the specific setting.

1.3   Theoretical perspectives

In the research literature on hospitalization theoretical explanations are seldom treated as central issues. This is understandable because hospitalization is a specific situation. Usually data are gathered to gauge the extent of the problems and to provide empirical foundations for practical solutions. Nevertheless, theory is useful or even necessary for effective prevention.

It is generally agreed that hospitalization is a stressful event for children and that subsequent disturbance is related to excessive stress (e.g., Moore, 1969; Nagera, 1978; Goslin, 1978 etc.). It has been demonstrated that children suffer because they fail to comprehend the change of surroundings, the nature of illness and the purpose of treatment. This is apparent from the ameliorating effects of preparation, for children of four years and older, which have already been discussed. Furthermore the fact that stress and risk of disturbance are related to age has been documented in many studies. Vulnerability increases steeply during the first year of life (Schaffer & Callender, 1959) and steadily decreases between the ages of three to four (Prugh et al., 1953; Vernon et al., 1965; Brain & Maclay, 1968; Douglas, 1975; Thompson, 1985). This fact is probably related to cognitive development and concomitant understanding of the situation. Equally important in connection with age is the emotional effect of separation of child/infant and attachment figures. The fact that rooming-in effects a considerable reduction of posthospital upset confirms the crucial impact of separation in this situation. Attachment theory provides an explanation for such an effect and a powerful basis for future research. The theoretical exposition to follow will articulate the relevance of stress research and of attachment theory in explaining posthospital upset and disturbance in children under three years of age. It is introduced by a summary.

A summary of theoretical explanation

Some children are unruffled by hospitalization and can even enjoy themselves. Also, for many children the staff of the ward may be a source of support. In spite of this, for *young* children that lack sufficient parental support, hospital treatment entails negative emotions, such as anxiety, fear, and depression. Such feelings in young children may be evoked by strange surroundings, strange people and uncomfortable or painful treatment. Sometimes these are superimposed on the discomfort of illness in itself. Such experiences and emotions are stressful, but the stress is not necessarily excessive. When stress is moderate the child may adapt to the situation. This is likely to happen when consistent support of parents is provided. There is a danger of later upset or disturbance when the amount of stress is excessive.

According to attachment theory a secure base for infants is represented by the parent or the caretaker to whom they are attached. Proximity to the attachment-figure has the capacity of buffering the effects of any external stressful circumstances. Her absence on the other hand has the effect of a steep increase in insecurity, because it means that the situation for the infant has become unpredictable and out of control. The natural consequence is an activation of the attachment behavioral system. This means that any action will be directed to regain proximity to the parent. Crying is the most common behavior under the circumstances. Depending on a number of conditions, of which duration of absence is primarily relevant, attachment behavior may ultimately be suppressed. Stress, however, may be undiminished while attachment behaviors are absent. The experience of a number of separation episodes can affect the attachment relationship. A few short (e.g., one night) separations are not usually sufficient to effect this change. Secure attachment can be transformed into avoidant attachment. Although separation may be a critical factor, the actual stress-experience is dependent on several other conditions. Security of the attachment relationship before hospitalization and sensitivity of the parents may modulate stress. External circumstances, such as restriction of movement will contribute to stressful experience.

Attachment theory by Bowlby

Attachment theory was conceived by Bowlby (1969) to clarify the ill effects of separation between infant and parents, formerly designated effects of maternal deprivation. A basic observation is the fact that human infants, similar to neonates of other species, develop a strong propensity to remain in the proximity of a specific adult: the attachment figure. The fylogenetic explanation employs the assumption that protection and survival is served by proximity; therefore behavioral systems in parent and infant promote proximity, especially in times of danger. The analogy to imprinting[1] in ducklings is explained in this fashion. Specific to humans, and consistent with the delayed maturity of human infants, is the fact that only in the second half of the first year the exclusive nature of attachment behaviors becomes manifest. Attachment behaviors will then be directed to one or several attachment figures, usually the mother or the parents. Examples of attachment behaviors are crying, clinging and early social interaction. While spatial proximity may be a sign of attachment, the function of the relationship is the enlistment of parental support. An important role is ascribed to the infant's confidence in his/her parent's accessibility and responsiveness. This will influence the distance experienced as safe and tolerance of short separations. Specific attachment behaviors will change with age. The functional role of the attachment behavioral system remains relatively unchanged while the child outgrows simple clinging behavior and progressively develops capacities for interaction over distance. The emotional tie between child and parent in later development will be the product of earlier attachment.

The attachment behavioral system is activated by distance or separation, but, in accordance with its origin, also by any sign of danger as apprehended by the infant, like strange people, discomfort, fatigue and illness. Compounding a strange environment, illness and separation produces the most powerful condition for attachment behavior. Exploratory behavior is inhibited by activation of the attachment behavioral system. Presence of an attachment figure as a secure base is a prerequisite to master a strange environment.

Bowlby (1969, 1973) describes three phases of response to prolonged separation. The first effect observed is a continuous activation of the attachment behavioral system: crying is a typical response, also the child will tend to seek the attachment figure or to wait for her reappearance. Substitute caregivers are often rejected. This is called the protest phase. If the attachment figure remains absent the protest will give way to a second phase with subdued or sad behavior, called the phase of despair. In a third phase the conspicuous emotional expression is reduced, the infant seems to be recovering from separation distress. Upon reunion, however, it is apparent that the relationship to the attachment figure has been seriously disrupted. Attachment behavior is absent in spite of the approach of the parent; the most salient response is a treatment of the attachment figure as if she were a complete stranger. This phase is called the

---

[1]   Newly hatched birds will approach any moving object and, even if this is not the true parent, henceforward maintain proximity to this object: "imprinting".

phase of detachment. Bowlby notes that the three phases of this sequence, first described by Robertson, are not sharply demarcated. The process described presupposes a rather prolonged separation, in the order of magnitude of at least several weeks. The full sequence, including detachment, will fortunately be exceptional in present clinical practice, although protest may often be observed.

It is a common observation that protest behavior can be absent for some time. The infant may sleep or be amenable to distraction by toys. Attachment behavior in the form of protest may reappear afterwards and the child may cry upon reunion, apparently releasing a suppressed emotional response. These observations are not contrary to the theory. Bowlby's concept of *defensive exclusion* is geared to explaining the absence of attachment behavior in situations where it might be expected (Bowlby, 1988). Defensive exclusion means that any stimulus or mental content tending to produce activation of the attachment behavioral system is obviated and excluded from consciousness, because of its painful nature. Bowlby envisages a full explanation of this possibility in terms of cognitive psychology, while he explicitly relates the concept to the Freudian notion of repression. Although his treatment seems to imply that defensive exclusion occurs in the phase of detachment, the same mechanism may be operative during separations of less than twelve hours. The discrepancy between overt behavior and actual stress experience, which has been documented by research on animals, can be misleading to observers, including caregivers.

The presence of attachment figures at critical times is important then in two different ways. The common assumption is that the infant needs care, support or reassurance and this is obviously true in various circumstances. The gist of attachment theory is that subjective security of the infant can be maintained by presence of the parent, even despite a stressful environment, while fundamental insecurity is engendered by separation despite adequate care. These basic principles are tested and confirmed by a plethora of empirical studies.

Security of attachment: the Ainsworth model

While some of the processes described above are fairly universal, even outside the boundary of our species, there are individual differences, which are of great importance for practical application. The development of some attachment relationship per se occurs independently of the quality of mothering (even in the case of maltreatment), but differences in quality of attachment have been demonstrated. In fact qualities of attachment have been the central issue of research into the beginnings of socio-emotional development for the last fifteen years. This trend in developmental psychology originates in the work of Mary Ainsworth, who devised a procedure to distinguish different patterns of attachment empirically: the well-known Strange Situation (Ainsworth & Wittig, 1969). This is a kind of individual experiment, performed for each mother-infant-dyad[2] separately, in a laboratory setting. The infant should not be much younger than one year old and not older than two. A strict protocol is supplied for the two adults, who interact with the child in this situation, the mother and a 'stranger' (an assistant). The mother is required to leave the child twice, for a few minutes. Because the surroundings are unfamiliar, the absence of the mother causes alarm for most children and attachment behavior is elicited. The sequence of events is videotaped and afterwards analyzed. Several aspects are important, particularly the behavior of the child towards the mother at the moment of reunion. Rating scales are employed for proximity seeking, maintaining physical contact, resistance to physical

---

[2]   For simplicity of exposition the mother is here referred to, while the father or another caregiver may be substituted.

contact and avoidance of the mother (Ainsworth, Blehar, Waters & Wall, 1978). Three categories of attachment quality have been established:

      type 'B': Secure attachment

      type 'A': Avoidant attachment: insecure

      type 'C': Ambivalent attachment: insecure.

The three categories are named here in the order of their frequency of occurrence in an ordinary population. Incidentally, it has been found that proportions may characteristically be influenced by patterns of culture (Van IJzendoorn & Tavecchio, 1987; Van IJzendoorn & Kroonenberg, 1988). Here we will just discuss the meaning of the three patterns of attachment in terms of behavior.[3] The emphasis is upon the behavior of the infant. It should be noted that the quality of attachment is not a property of the infant; the behavior of a 'type X infant' is actually the behavior of an infant in the context of a type X attachment relationship. The infant may behave differently toward another attachment figure. Most of the research data pertain to the infant-mother attachment relationship.

Type B infants are positive in their behavior towards the attachment figure; the phrase 'a secure base' is most apt for this category. Their attachment behavioral system is well-tuned: it is not aroused without sufficient reason and its activation is properly terminated by consolation by the mother. This is apparent in the Strange Situation. Furthermore, infants deemed to have secure attachments are found to be more positively outgoing and cooperative with playmates and even with relatively unfamiliar adults. Origins of secure attachment are sought in early mother-infant interaction. The contribution of the mother, commonly conceived as sensitive responsiveness will be discussed later.

Type A infants are conspicuous for their avoidant behavior in the reunion episodes of the Strange Situation, a moment when attachment behavior is theoretically expected to be manifest at highest intensity. Avoidance in this context means that the infant fails to approach the mother, or that an initial approach is interrupted. Also characteristic, and thought to be revealing of the underlying mechanism, is aversion of the gaze. The meaning of this behavior is carefully interpreted by Main (1977) and Ainsworth et al. (1978), in connection with the finding that type A-infants had experienced rejection by their mothers, at least in the sense that these mothers were disinclined or even averse to cuddling their infant. Type A mothers are described as rigid and compulsive. Their children are supposed to have a normal need for close bodily contact, but to be caught in an approach-avoidance conflict. Avoidance is a way to reduce excessive arousal resulting from this conflict and leaves the situation open to the possibility of subsequent positive interaction. Of course it is not assumed that the infant consciously conceives of such a strategy. It seems to be consistent with the aforementioned interpretations, as well as with the ideas of Bowlby, to consider avoidant behavior as a product of repeated episodes of defensive exclusion, resulting from failed interaction within the context of attachment. Such failure may be related to the personality of the mother, alternatively temporary absence during episodes of severe distress, or a kind of helplesness at the time of critical events (painful treatment) may have the same effect. Stressful situations have been implicated as possible precursors of a shift from secure to insecure attachment (Riksen-Walraven, 1983). Defensive exclusion in Bowlby's terms may occur in such cases and may eventually develop into a pattern of avoidant response. A logical consequence is the hypothesis that hospitalization with insufficient parental presence may cause an increase in avoidant attachment.

Type C infants are called ambivalent or resistant because the infant tends to exhibit a mixture of approach and resistant behavior in bodily contact with the attachment figure. The

---

[3]   The classification system has been recently extended by some authors with a fourth category D: Disorganized, insecure. The validity of this extension requires further study (Van IJzendoorn et al., 1991).

infants are chronically anxious in relation to the mother, therefore the mother's departure provokes severe distress. Their attachment behavioral system appears to have a low threshold for high intensity activation, a pattern which may also be termed excessive separation anxiety. In contrast to infants with a secure attachment relationship they fail to be comforted quickly or thoroughly when their mother returns. Anger and the need for comfort produce ambivalent behavior. The cause of this interaction pattern is apparently a lack of responsive behavior, or a lack of consistency in responding on the part of the attachment figure. In contrast to type A dyads there is no evidence of an attitude of rejection on the part of mothers in a type C dyad. In hospital situations the stress is likely to be severe for type C infants.

Hospitalization and subsequent quality of attachment

The hypothesis that hospitalization could be conducive to type A attachments was introduced above. Three studies are available on the effect of illness and/or hospitalization on quality of attachment. Although these have been conducted from the more general notion that chronic illness or hospitalization will affect security of attachment, they tend to confirm this more specific hypothesis.

Fischer-Fay, Goldberg, Simmons and Levison (1988) obtained attachment classifications for twenty-three infants with cystic fibrosis and an equal number of matched controls. The average age was fifteen months; the chronically ill infants had spent an average of three weeks in hospital. Of infants with cystic fibrosis 35% was classified as avoidant as opposed to 20% of controls, but differences were not significant.

Gotowiecz, Fischer-Fay and Morris (1990) compared three groups of children at the age of one year: 24 infants with congenital heart disease, 13 with cystic fibrosis and 33 healthy controls. They report a significant difference between controls and children with a heart disease, confirming less secure attachments among chronically ill infants. They omit data on hospitalization. On closer scrutiny their data support our hypothesis with 10% type A relationships among healthy controls, 24% among infants with cystic fibrosis and 46% among those with congenital heart disease, while differences in proportions of ambivalent attachment are slight.

Hoeksma and Koomen (1991) studied infants with cleft lip and palate and controls in the 10-18 months developmental stage. From their experimental design it can be concluded that avoidant behavior in a stressful situation at home as well as in the Strange Situation is significantly increased after recent hospital experiences. In a recently hospitalized subgroup 50% of twelve infants was classified as avoidant, but due to the size of the groups the overall difference in security classifications was short of significance. The Hoeksma & Koomen data suggest that an increase in avoidant behavior may diminish or disappear after a number of months.

As suggested in our exposition, a causal explanation linking avoidant behavior to hospitalization is likely, while a more direct link between illness and avoidant behavior is difficult to specify theoretically. Van IJzendoorn, Goldberg, Kroonenberg and Frenkel (1992) performed a meta-analysis concerning the effect of various types of obstacles on the development of secure attachment. It was concluded that maternal problems, such as mental illness, clearly affect quality of attachment, whereas infant problems, such as deafness or Down's syndrome, did not produce significantly abnormal attachment classifications. The effect of hospitalization was not considered here. The data compiled by Van IJzendoorn et al. indicates that a normal (U.S.A.) population comprises 20% type A cases ($N = 1584$). If the hospitalized samples from the three studies cited here are pooled, a rate of 39% ($N = 72$) is found, a definite increase (*Chi square* is 13.9, $df = 1$, $p < .001$).[4]

Hospitalization and stress

To prevent oversimplification it should be emphasized that the adverse effects of hospitalization are not dependent on any specific event, but on the psychological meaning of events for particular subjects. Absence of attachment figures may be a critical event for one infant because it is experienced as rejection, whereas another infant appreciates the facts in a different way. The distress of separation is moreover modified by other sources of discomfort.

Stress can be defined as the responses of the body to a variety of noxious stimuli or emotional experiences. These responses constitute a syndrome involving activation of the pituitary-adrenal system, which has been the focus of a whole body of research. We suggest that events are traumatic when the subject is no longer able to cope with the situation and that the notions of stress and coping, while congenial to most theoretical explanations, are not, in this context, tautological and therefore redundant. This conviction is strengthened by neuroendocrine indices for intensity of stressful experience. The results acquired in this fashion are consistent with attachment-theoretical propositions.

Stress may be a 'fact of life' and an essential ingredient in learning, which usually means: attaining some sort of control in the given situation. Löschenkohl (1981) speaks of 'Umweltbewältigung' as the main challenge for four-year-olds in a hospital situation. If such coping is feasible, then stress can have a steeling effect (Garmezy, 1983) and prepare the subject for later similar experience, a process closely akin to immunization (Damsté, 1981). If not, the stress may be excessive and the vulnerability of the subject increased, which will show itself in behavioral disturbances. This course of events is traumatic. Such general notions are valuable, in spite of the fact that they can not be readily tested by any particular empirical study.

Knight et al. (1979) investigated the neuro-endocrine responses of nineteen 7-11 year old children admitted to hospital for minor surgery. The assumption that emotional distress, observable on a behavioral level would be reflected in metabolites of ACTH was confirmed. More important, it was demonstrated that effectiveness in coping, judged by clinical and projective techniques could reduce stress, as measured by cortisol secretion in urine samples. Furthermore 'ward adjustment' proved to be significantly related to cortisol production. Similar data pertaining to human *infants* are not available, but research on animals provides additional perspective.

Levine (1983) in his review of a number of studies relevant to 'the ontogeny of coping' documents that *loss of control* proves to be the most potent source of distress among a large variety of experimental conditions. According to his theoretical viewpoint separation of infants from their mother represents for the infant unmitigated loss of control. Any mastery over the environment and it's stimulus patterns is acquired within the context of early attachment. The convergence with the theories of Bowlby is bolstered by stress-research on monkeys. In infant squirrel monkeys a vigorous endocrine response to separation was obtained in both infant and mother after thirty minutes. After six hours of separation the stress for infants was observed to be higher, judging by plasma cortisol values, than in any other experimental situation. This was particularly revealing because protest behavior, that had reached a peak shortly after the separation procedure, had been considerably reduced after six hours. This situation can

---

[4]   Available studies, cited by Van IJzendoorn et al. (1992) concerning clinical samples with a problem of prematurity are deliberately not included in this comparison.

theoretically be described by stating that despair may be manifest after only a few hours. Equivalently, it may be argued that protest behavior is suppressed, since it has proved to be meaningless for the subject, and the stage has been set for intra-organismic defence, like 'defensive exclusion'.

Buffering of stress for infants and mothers, so long as they remain in each other's presence, appeared to be a fitting explanation for several experimental findings. In monkey dyads this was demonstrated by pseudo-separations. Mother and infant were caught, removed from their home cage and separated by force, a procedure eliciting violent protest. When they were reunited immediately, this procedure failed to elicit a neuroendocrine response, presumably because no actual separation had been effected.

An experiment involving substitute care is also relevant for the situation of human infants in hospital. Here monkey infants were provided with the opportunity of clinging to a substitute mother (a late pregnant female) when their mothers were removed, a kind of behavior absent under normal conditions. It seemed that this emergency solution was effective, because behavioral agitation of the infants was significantly reduced. Measurements of plasma cortisol, however, demonstrated that the stress for infants in this situation was similar to that during separations where 'aunting' was precluded. In the same vein, while behavioral distress could be reduced by objects like a cloth-mother, the intensity of upset was undiminished (Levine, 1983).

After this excursion into animal research we will not omit the customary note of caution regarding the validity of experimental findings on animals for human experience and behavior. It is striking, however, that results should agree so well. In sum: it appears that stress (engendered by hospitalization) is chemically measurable and this sensitive index for emotional experience should alert us to the fact that behavioral indices are sometimes misleading. It should be especially noted that, although protest behavior may be absent, the separation from attachment figures can still cause distress. The design of our present study does not include measurement of neuroendocrine secretion, but a theory to explain behavioral disturbance must include the concept of stress.

Attachment quality and sensitivity as modifiers

Two constructs of parent-child interaction have been identified as relevant: Security of attachment and sensitivity as a contribution of the parent to the relationship. It is not far-fetched to hypothesize that stress and risk of disturbance will be less in the case of secure attachment. The securely attached infant will presumably be less fearful, more cooperative towards a physician or nurse and less easily distressed by short separations, either in the daytime or during the night.

Sensitivity is frequently defined as the caregiver's awareness of the specific needs of the infant in various situations and her ability to respond appropriately. It may not be assumed a priori that sensitivity as it is measured will predict quality of attachment. In fact, although the early study of Ainsworth and associates reported a strong connection (Ainsworth et al., 1978), a number of studies have failed to confirm this result. Although inconsistencies between research outcomes are common, a meta-analysis by Goldsmith and Alansky (1987), demonstrated that measured sensitivity accounted for a modest part of differences in security of attachment. In her recent review of twenty eight studies concerning the relationship between maternal behavior and subsequent attachment quality, Lambermon (1991) arrived at the same conclusion. Therefore it is presumed that maternal sensitivity can ameliorate stress in the hospital in one or both of two different ways. It may contribute to a secure initial attachment relationship and it may account for better parental support during critical events in the hospital. It is important to evaluate the effects of parental presence in hospital without confounding presence and sensitivity. Both aspects of parental support will be examined in the prospective study.

1.4   Summing up

It has been established by several decades of research that the socio-emotional development of young infants may be affected by hospital treatment, depending on a number of conditions. For the majority of children in hospital no serious problems are to be expected, because they are no longer of the most sensitive age, not staying more than one or a few days, not readmitted at an early age, not severely hurt or restricted in freedom by treatment, and/or not left without parental support for a substantial amount of time. British studies of long-term effects have suggested that, if adverse conditions prevail, emotional scars may remain for any number of years. These studies are presumably outdated as regards the prevalence of such unfavorable conditions, especially the absence of attachment figures in the hospital. It must be admitted however, that the effects of present day policy for patients who are at risk is unknown.

For a theoretical explanation it is proposed here that hospital experience may become traumatic if the degree of stress in the hospital situation is felt to be beyond any available coping mechanism. It may sooner be experienced as such when attachment figures, usually parents, are inaccessible. On the other hand, if the situation is found to be manageable the tolerance for future admissions may become enhanced. Initial secure attachment is hypothesized to be a protective factor. The crucial protection is considered to be parental support during the hospital experience. This support factor can be decomposed into parental sensitivity and parental attendance. Finally, the hypothesis is discussed that the hospitalization experience may entail damage to the quality of the attachment relationship between child and caregiver. In particular it may occur that secure attachment gives way to avoidant attachment. This idea is supported by data of three empirical studies into attachment quality between chronically ill infants and their mothers.

The effect of conditions that are presumed important here has been investigated and tested in the two studies that are the substance of this book. The first is a small-sample retrospective project, reported completely in Chapter 2. The second is an elaborate experimental prospective study of 64 surgical patients and their families. It will be reported in Chapters 3 to 7. For readers only interested in the prospective study it is a possibility to skip the next chapter and continue with Chapter 3. Final results will be aggregated and integrated in the final chapter.

CHAPTER 2   THE PRELIMINARY RETROSPECTIVE STUDY

This chapter is concerned with the retrospective study, originally an extended pilot study. The *prospective* pilot (Fahrenfort, Jacobs & Kaptein- de Kock van Leeuwen, 1990) will not be reported explicitly in this volume, because it has only served as a stepping stone for the design of the major study described in Chapters 3 to 6. The *retrospective* study, on the other hand, has been extended in order to yield independent substantive data.

Section 2.1 describes the purpose and hypotheses, Section 2.2 the method. Sections 2.3 and 2.4 give the results of the first and of the second analysis. The results are discussed in Section 2.5.

2.1 Introduction

The retrospective approach was considered useful because it allowed (a) sampling of subjects according to hospitalization history and (b) a period of several years for follow-up. As a point of departure the following hypotheses were formulated:

I   Children experiencing *prolonged or repeated* hospitalization during the 6-36 months developmental stage run a serious risk of developmental damage, manifest in behavior for several years.

II   The extent of problematic behavior in the population referred to will be associated with number of admissions and length of hospitalization.

III   Several modes of parental care in hospital, like daily availability of parents and rooming-in can prevent later behavior disturbance.

IV   Problems during the first months after discharge will reflect the quality of parental support in hospital and predict future disequilibrium.

These hypotheses are consistent with the theory considered in the first chapter, without, however, representing the nuances of attachment theory. Some expected consequences can be tested by a retrospective design, attributing validity to a family's report concerning (a) parental presence in the hospital, (b) behavior of the infant shortly after discharge and (c) behavior problems at the time of data collection.

2.2 Method

Procedure and subjects

Three Dutch hospitals have contributed to the study: the 'Diaconessenhuis' Leiden, the 'Merwede Hospital' Dordrecht, and the 'University Hospital Leiden'. 65 Children were selected from hospital records dating from 1-1-1986 onward. Selection was based on the hospitalization history of children admitted at least once in the sensitive age-range of 6-36 months. The rationale of sampling was to acquire an unrestricted cross-section of the population of children with this specific kind of experience, the experience predating data collection at least several years. No restrictions were put on the diagnosis or treatment, except that it should be 'somatic'. Such a strategy is rather different from the sampling in the prospective study which was limited to surgical medicine.

In order to obtain a considerable variety of hospitalization histories, selection was performed according to the following criteria:
- specific selection of multiple admissions in the (sensitive) 6-36 months period;
- specific selection of cases with long term single admissions;
- no early admissions in the 0-6 months period, thus deliberately excluding cases of premature birth;
- no admissions after 36 months (as far as recorded in the same hospital);
- exclusion of chronically hospitalized children.

Families (n = 65) were approached by mail via the hospitals with a request to participate. Those who responded positively (n = 44) received and returned questionnaires. These we call the original sample. The sample included cases of general pediatrics, general pediatric surgery, ophtalmology, heart surgery, and neurology. A small subset of the sample (n = 15) was visited at home for additional information: the subsample.

A control group was recruited from the younger pupils of three elementary schools in different towns in The Netherlands. For this purpose 191 families were approached by mail.

121 Questionnaires were returned. For the sake of comparison between sample and control-group a selection was made from each group as reported in Section 2.3.

Questionnaires and instruments

Questions on the circumstances of hospitalization and the child's behavior afterwards at home were addressed to families of the hospitalized sample. On the subject of parental presence and participation no questionnaire was available. A number of questions was designed; these questions are reproduced in Appendix 1.

The topics were:
PQ3. the parental share in non-medical care like washing, and feeding;
PQ4. contribution of play-leaders;
PQ5. regulation of visiting hours;
PQ6. the extent of mother's presence during the day;
PQ7. the extent of father's presence during the day;
PQ8. degree of physical pain judged by parents;
PQ9. rooming-in, opportunity and actual practice;
PQ10. presence at anaesthesia induction.

As can be seen, the items concerning involvement of parents were interspersed with other subjects, for example the question relating to physical pain. These questions were added as dummy questions, to reduce the emphasis on the subject of parental presence. A scale for parental attendance was constructed on the basis of PQ3, PQ4, PQ6, PQ7, PQ9 and PQ10. An itemscore for PQ4 was assigned according to the knowledge of parents about any contribution by play-leaders; parents who reported ignorance on the subject obtained a lower score. Coefficient alpha for this pool of six items was found to be .63. This figure was not very satisfactory. All item-total correlations were positive, however, and no items were discarded.

Nine items were constructed to assess symptoms of upset during the first months after discharge. Items were common behavior disorders after hospitalization, for instance: "Did your child (at the time) have trouble either going to bed or to sleep?" (cf. Appendix 1). The report of Douglas (1975) suggested that such retrospective information might have predictive value. Because we had to rely on the memory of parents only simple clear-cut topics were included. The scale was called *REA: Short-term response to hospitalization*. Coefficient alpha was computed as .75. All items were retained.

BCL: Behavior Checklist

Questions on current behavior were addressed to sample and control-group alike. The BCL, the principal measure of present behavioral problems employed here, was developed by Richman, Stevenson and Graham (1982). This is the written questionnaire version of the Behaviour Screening Questionnaire (BSQ), designed for epidemiological research on childhood disorders. The BSQ is discussed at length in Chapter 3 and 4. Validity studies were satisfactory for the BSQ (Earls, Jacobs, Goldfein & Silbert, 1982; Swets-Gronert, 1986) and the BCL (Richman, 1977). Three items were added, specifically for five year olds, as most research using the list has been conducted in samples of three year olds, whereas the present age range is wider. BCL-scores were obtained of both hospitalized and non-hospitalized subjects. The score was computed in standard fashion by simple addition. Coefficient alpha was .72.

Ego-Resilience.

The 15 families visited at home completed the NCKS (Nijmegen-California Kinder Sorteer Techniek) a Dutch version of the California Child Q-set (CCQ), (Block & Block, 1980; Van Lieshout, Riksen-Walraven, Ten Brink et al., 1986). Among the traits that can be measured 'Ego-resilience' is a particular useful index for socio-emotional adaptation. This trait refers to flexibility and persistence in problem solving exhibited in various situations. The concept has acquired a firm construct validity in the research cited above.

Primary and secondary analysis

In a first analysis, preceding the prospective study, the possible association of hospitalization history and problem behavior was investigated by a comparison between children with and without hospitalization history. Furthermore, after constructing scales for parental attendance (PQ) and for short-term response after discharge (REA), correlations were computed within the sample.

In a secondary analysis, after completion of the prospective study, the ANCOVA-approach of the latter was utilized to reconsider the relevance of some items concerning conditions of hospitalization, especially parental attendance. This secondary analysis should be regarded as exploratory, as opposed to hypothesis-testing.

2.3　Results of primary analysis

Outline of parental support in the original sample (1986)

BASIC CARE: Of 44 parents in the original sample (mostly mothers) 22 reported that basic care, like feeding and bathing was provided mainly by themselves. Three mothers had transferred such care to the nursing staff; 19 had chosen intermediate solutions.

PRESENCE DURING DAYTIME: The majority, 29, reported extensive presence at daytime with a minimum of 5 hours. Some were continuously present. Ten mothers reported a presence of 3-5 hours and five a presence of less than 3 hours.

ROOMING-IN: Only a minority of 11 parents did provide such care. In 7 cases rooming-in was not allowed. Answers of parents concerning this question:

rooming-in was unnecessary	8
rooming-in was not possible	11
parents were lodged in a separate room	2
at least one night of rooming-in	5
every night rooming-in	6
not relevant (one day admission)	2

PRESENCE AT INDUCTION OF ANAESTHESIA: Of 21 children undergoing surgery, 8 children were accompanied by one of the parents during induction of anaesthesia.

Reported symptoms of short-term upset by retrospective report (N = 44)

Symptoms of upset during the first three months after discharge (REA-items) were reported in many cases. The following problems, arranged in descending frequency were either serious or transient:

waking up at night	47%
afraid to be alone in a room	41%
management problems	36%
fussy about bedtime	34%
angry, aggressive	23%
subdued	18%
need for pedagogical help	9%

In the last category, need for pedagogical help, two families were included who sought professional advice and two families who did not, but reported this need in our survey.

Sample description and selection

I SELECTION WITHIN THE SAMPLE: On the basis of previous findings (Douglas, 1975; Davenport & Werry, 1970) no long-term effects were attributed to hospitalization lasting only a few days. Therefore it was decided to count a 'hospitalization history' of three days or less as no hospitalization history. The sample included two such cases, that were consequently excluded from the comparison.

A minor problem was the relevance of two cases, because of the extra information supplied by the parents. This information was prompted by our request to add anything that might be important, but could not be covered by the questionnaires. In one case the first admission was provoked by problem behavior, thus confounding the criterion. And in the second case the family situation had evidently been severely disturbing. This young boy moreover was extreme on three of the relevant variables: he obtained the highest scores on hospitalization history and behavioral difficulties and the lowest score on parental attendance during hospitalization. Although reasons might be advanced for including the case of the boy, it was judged more cautious to exclude both. Thus the sample was reduced by four exclusions to fourty cases.

II SELECTION WITHIN THE CONTROL-GROUP: Obviously cases with a hospitalization history of longer than three days had to be removed from the control-group. Such cases constituted the group of hospitalized controls. Furthermore, in order to balance the mean age of the two selected groups, only children older than four years of age were chosen as selected controls. The selected control-group consisted of 73 cases. A description of the groups for age can be found in Table 2.1. A comparison for hospitalization history is provided by Table 2.2. The original sample is included in this table to illustate the selection process.

TABLE 2.1   *Age and time elapsed after latest recorded discharge until the time of the data collection*

age in months	M	(SD)	range
unselected controls (n = 121)	54	(9)	33 - 75
selected sample (n = 40)	59	(6)	38 - 74
selected controls (n = 73)	58	(7)	49 - 75
hospitalized controls (n = 15)	55	(8)	42 - 69
time elapsed	M	(SD)	range
selected sample (n = 40)	36	(10)	13 - 52

TABLE 2.2   *Hospitalization history, descriptive statistics*

frequency of recorded admissions	M	(SD)	range
original sample (n = 44)	2.4	(2.0)	1 - 9
selected sample (n = 40)	2.4	(2.0)	1 - 9
selected controls (n = 73)	.2	(.4)	0 - 2
hospitalized controls (n = 15)	1.6	(1.0)	1 - 4
accumulated hospital days	M	(SD)	range
original sample (n = 44)	21.1	(20.7)	1 - 88
selected sample (n = 40)	20.4	(18.4)	5 - 79
selected controls (n = 73)	.3	(.8)	0 - 3
hospitalized controls (n = 15)	11.3	(10.2)	4 - 42

Hospitalization history and current problem behavior

A comparison of the sample *with* hospitalization history and the controls *without* shows a significant difference in scores for problem behavior in favor of the controls. The t-test is displayed in Table 2.3. This finding tends to support the hypothesis that disturbances due to hospitalization may persist for years in a number of cases. To rule out the remote possibility that the origin of the groups might contribute to the difference by factors other than hospitalization, a comparison is made between controls without hospitalization history and hospitalized controls. Although there is only a handful of hospitalized controls, the expected difference is once more found to be significant.

TABLE 2.3   *Behavior problem scores for children with and without hospitalization history*

		BCL-scores		one-sided	
	n	*M*	*(SD)*	*t*	*p*
selected sample	40	8.0	(3.9)		
selected controls	73	6.7	(3.9)	1.67*	.048
hospitalized controls	15	9.3	(4.7)		
selected controls	73	6.7	(3.9)	1.96*	.033

* indicates a t-value significant at the .05 level

For individual BCL-items t-values are not reproduced, because a multiple t-test for the items requires a Bonferroni correction which is not a realistic standard in our small sample. The most discriminating items referred to the following difficulties:
  - poor concentration
  - attention seeking
  - soiling
  - fearfulness

The Pearson correlations within the selected sample are displayed in Table 2.4. They provide little support for the hypotheses presented in the introduction. Principal findings are:
- The correlation between hospital-days and BCL confirms the difference just obtained. When all subjects available are pooled this correlation is found to be .25 (n = 165; p = .001).
- All correlations of parental attendance with measures of later adjustment are insignificant.
- The short-term response as measured here is unrelated to any other variable.
- The correlation of -.81 between BCL and ego-resilience offers a satisfactory confirmation of concurrent validity.

TABLE 2.4   *Pearson correlations within the selected sample*

	2	3	4	5	6
1. accumulated h-days	.51*	-.05	-.21	.27*	-.27
2. admission frequency		-.00	.16	.22	-.25
3. REA: short-term response			.17	.11	.15
4. PQ: parental attendance				-.10	.41
5. BCL: behavior problems					-.81*
6. ego-resilience (n=15)					

for ego-resilience n = 15; for parental attendance n = 39 because of one missing value; otherwise n = 40.
* is printed where p < .05 , one-sided.

2.4 Secondary analysis

It appears from the correlation with ego-resilience that the BCL-scores are valid. The provisional retrospective assessment of short-term upset after discharge is, considered in retrospect, inadequate. The question remains whether the information about parental attendance should be rejected or respected. We do not expect this information about simple facts to be grossly distorted by the passage of time. Social desirability may be a source of bias. The scaling did present problems. The internal consistency was unsatisfactory, a reason to distrust the scale, rather than the answers. The items on presence of mother and presence of father in hospital had the disadvantage that no estimate was obtained of the time covered by means of alternate caretaking. Such reflections prompted a renewed analysis, where information from single questions was tested for possible predictive value. The criterion is once more the BCL-score at the time of data collection. The technique is analysis of covariance, a statistical method that will be explained and dicussed in Section 5.1.

The first predictor is the fact of surgery. Surgery was performed on 21 of 40 children in the selected sample. At the time of the first analysis it had already been detected that their problem behavior scores were elevated. The difference in means is shown in Table 2.5. An ANCOVA was executed with hospital-days as a covariate. The *F*-value, reported in Table 2.6 indicates a significant disadvantage for the surgical category, which applies irrespective of differences in amount of hospitalization. Henceforward both hospital-days and surgery were systematically entered as covariates.
Non-medical care was distinguished as 'mainly' provided by the parent or partially/completely by the staff. Parental care implicated a lower mean for eventual BCL-scores, but when adjustment was made for both covariates the difference was not significant (Table 2.6).

The other two items of parental attendance, daily presence (by mother) and rooming-in (by father or mother), do not significantly predict later development. Surprisingly, a significant difference of behavior is predicted by two items, previously treated as 'dummy questions': play-leader sessions and pain during treatment retrospectively reported by parents.

TABLE 2.5   *Descriptive statistics of BCL for a number of single-item predictors (n = 39)*

item:	n	M	(SD)
surgery:			
yes	21	9.5	(4.3)
no	19	6.4	(3.0)
non-medical care:			
mainly by parent/mother	19	7.2	(3.5)
otherwise	20	8.8	(4.5)
maternal daily presence:			
at least five hours	23	7.8	(3.6)
less	16	8.3	(4.8)
rooming-in:			
at least one night	10	7.0	(4.2)
not at all	29	8.4	(4.0)
play-leader sessions:			
yes	21	6.5	(2.1)
no (or unknown)	18	9.8	(4.9)
pain (by parent-report):			
no severe pain	24	7.0	(3.4)
severe pain	15	9.7	(4.6)

TABLE 2.6   *Surgery, parental attendance and additional items as predictors (n = 39)*

item:	F	(df)	p
surgery	11.0	(1,37)	.003
parental care	1.1	(1,36)	.298
maternal presence	.8	(1,36)	.379
rooming-in	.1	(1,36)	.820
play-sessions	6.0	(1,36)	.020
pain (parent-report)	3.3	(1,36)	.080

covariate for surgery is hospital-days; for the other items covariates are hospital-days and surgery.

2.5   Discussion

Some weaknesses of the study are obvious. The non-response is considerable: about 30% among those selected for hospitalization history, which may have influenced results. Doubts about validity of some independent variables could not be eliminated; for this reason Hypothesis IV, concerning problems during the first months after discharge, could not be tested adequately.

The data have convincingly demonstrated that an increase of behavior problems is related to a history of hospitalization. The point is that for children in the sample hospitalization and surgery have occurred several years ago, as reflected in Table 2.1. A period of several years in this developmental stage represents nearly half a lifetime and considerable opportunity to readjust. It is justified to speak of a developmental disturbance of those concerned. In view of the history of the problem and the theoretical knowledge in this field it is reasonable to ascribe such disturbance primarily to hospitalization. In some cases, however, the illness may have contributed in other ways that can not be distinguished in our data.

A number of circumstances or parameters of hospitalization have been studied for their predictive value. The total of hospital-days appeared to be a weak but consistent predictor. This is consistent with the plausible assumption that other factors co-determine outcomes. Frequency is not a good predictor, but because of its relationship to hospital-days, remains a relevant parameter. Hypothesis III, which suggests that parental attendance is a crucial condition to prevent or to reduce traumatic experience has not been confirmed. The secondary analysis makes it unlikely that scaling problems are responsible for this result; it can be interpreted to mean that the importance of parental attendance has been overestimated in the theoretical treatment. This inference remains doubtful, however, in view of the limitations of the study. Among other objections, it should be noted that full rooming-in was insufficiently practiced to judge the benefits.

The analysis hints that events and conditions during hospitalization, such as surgery and pain, modify experience and later adjustment. The impact of surgery seems to be strong: this finding is convincing, even if unpredicted. The relationship of BCL-scores to pain as reported retrospectively by parents is interesting and remarkable, but it is only an exploratory result. The reduced incidence of behavior problems among children who were reported to have been engaged in sessions with the play-leader is ambiguous: these children may have benefitted from play activities, but may also have suffered less serious health problems.

The most important general conclusion is that adverse effects of hospitalization may persist for years if conditions are unfavorable, as they are for a minority of children. Behavioral manifestations are only a trace of traumatic experience. The results confirm the relevance of attempts to prevent such outcomes. For this purpose a different research design will now be described: that of the larger and more complicated prospective study.

CHAPTER 3   METHOD OF THE PROSPECTIVE INVESTIGATION

Chapter 3 contains a description of the purpose and design of the study. Hypotheses that should be tested are stated in Section 3.1. The hypothetical influence of some constructs on the adjustment of the child is visually displayed in Figure 3.1. Formal characteristics of the population and specifications of the sample can be found in Section 3.2. For a full description of the sample the reader should consult Section 4.1 as well. The design is presented in Section 3.3, including specifications of instruments and the sequence of measurements. Figure 3.2 provides a summary of such information. The interventions, their rationale and substance, are described in Section 3.4.

3.1   General outline

Purpose

Our research is designed to detect developmental disturbances in infants and toddlers caused by hospitalization, including surgery, under present (1990-1991) conditions in The Netherlands. It is a short-term longitudinal investigation, where assessment of disturbance occurs one month, two months and at least nine months after discharge. Posthospital behavior problems during the first six weeks after discharge are classified as *psychological upset*. They are presumed to be transient unless they can be demonstrated as persisting. A child can be considered to suffer from *developmental disturbance* if several behavioral symptoms (as measured by the Behavior Screening Questionnaire described in 3.1) outlast the first few months after hospitalization; thus problems after two months are possible symptoms of disturbance and continuous problems after nine months are definite symptoms of disturbance.

Impairment of educational achievement has been found by Douglas (1975) and Haslum (1988). Hypothetically, hospitalized infants may become delayed in language and speech development, either because of emotional factors or independent of them. This aspect is covered by screening language and speech development in the final follow up.

A principal objective of the study is to investigate the feasibility of prevention by encouraging parental involvement. Interventions intending to promote presence of parents in the hospital and adequate support of infants are directed towards an experimental group comprising a randomly selected half of the total sample.

Hypotheses

Past research and common sense suggest that upset or disturbance will in general be associated with number and duration of hospital admissions. Many infants in the sample have sustained multiple admissions. If early hospitalization can produce long-lasting disturbance this should be apparent in their present preadmission adjustment scores. Posthospital adjustment on the other hand should best be predicted by the interaction of the length of admission with the adequacy of parental support. Beyond this basic premiss, it is hypothesized that parental support, including presence and sensitive parenting can be enhanced by intervention. The following hypotheses include these general and a number of more specific propositions, provided by our theoretical discussion.

(1)   Prehospital adjustment will be related to hospitalization history: frequency and duration of preceding hospital admissions.

(2)   Adequate adjustment in spite of hospital experience indicates decreased or low vulnerability; prehospital maladjustment indicates increased vulnerability.

(3)   Interventions directed towards the parents will effect better parental support.
Enhancement of parental support may be manifest as:
- longer presence at daytime in the hospital
- more frequent rooming-in at night
- more frequent presence at induction of anaesthesia
- more involvement of fathers

(4)   Posthospital upset and maladjustment will be reduced by interventions.

(5)   Posthospital adjustment will be related to the duration of a new admission.

(6)   Posthospital adjustment will be related to parental support; parental presence and sensitivity.

(7)   Quality of attachment will modify posthospital adjustment; maladjustment will be more likely when attachment is insecure.

(8)   Duration of admission and parental presence will exhibit interactional effects.

(9)   Insufficient parental presence in hospital will disturb the child-caregiver relationship, specifically increase avoidant behavior.

(10)   Developmental disturbance will be related to the same predictors as short-term upset.

(11)   Speech or language acquisition will be related to the same predictors as posthospital adjustment.

At present a full discussion of interrelationships among predictors will be omitted, although this subject will require attention in the statistical analysis. A diagrammatic model of possible influences conceived of in the theory is provided in Figure 3.1 (p. 47). The presumed interactions of predictors involved in their effects on stress and maladjustment are not represented in this figure. In fact, the model does not claim to provide an exhaustive account of causal interactions and statistical associations. Such a model would entail speculation that could hardly be transformed into useful knowledge, even in the future. The present model serves as a summary of hypotheses and a symbol of their theoretical connectedness. A survey of measurements pertaining to the general concepts employed here is provided in Figure 3.2 (p. 53).

FIGURE 3.1. *Factors theoretically predicting posthospital maladjustment*

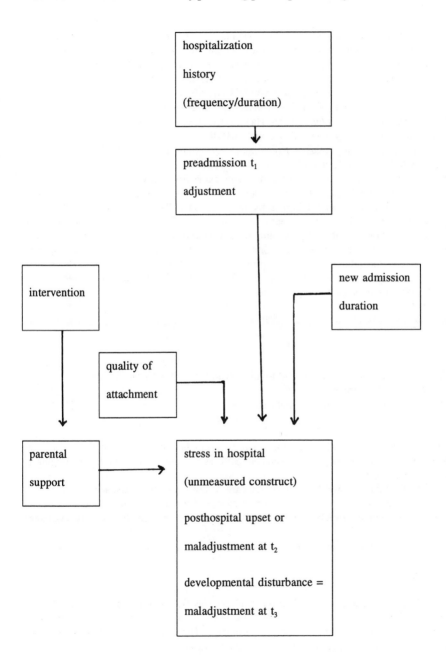

3.2   Hospitals and subjects

Participating hospitals

Because adjustment of infant patients and their parents may be influenced by the hospital staff, the environment and the policy within hospitals, it was decided to seek participation by a number of different hospitals. Cooperation was requested from and granted by six hospitals:

AZL, *Academisch Ziekenhuis Leiden*, a large University Hospital

AZVU, *Academisch Ziekenhuis van de Vrije Universiteit*
(University Hospital of the Free University) in Amsterdam

JKZ, *Juliana Kinderziekenhuis* in Den Haag, a Children's Hospital

Reinier de Graaf, a large General Hospital in Delft

SKZ, *Sophia Kinderziekenhuis* in Rotterdam, a University Hospital for Children

St Clara Ziekenhuis, a General Hospital in Rotterdam

Because of restrictions on the sample most participants came from university hospitals and from the JKZ. Spotting of eligible patients was mostly done by the admission department or by a secretary on the children's ward, sometimes by the physician. The official was regularly and frequently approached by the research team for new cases. The responsible physician was contacted to inquire about possible impediments to involve the family. Such impediments could be the expressly formulated restrictions on the population or, in rare cases, specific circumstances like a hospitalization history too extensive to allow for a remotely normal development. The usual course would be that the physician notified parents of the research. If parents had no objections to discussing the matter, the researcher would inform the parents on the research protocol and obtain their cooperation, or refusal.

Subjects: the population

The population was restricted to infants and toddlers with the following characteristics.

(1) age: 12 to 36 months

(2) surgical intervention (with full anaesthesia)

(3) expected to stay for at least seven hospital days

(4) no *severe* mental handicap

For practical reasons families where communication would be difficult or impossible for the research team, because of language were excluded. Still, as intended, some families belonging to ethnic minorities participated.

Although it seemed desirable to study any case of hospitalization expected to last a week or longer, in the main study recruitment was restricted to surgical cases. This precluded cases of hospitalization motivated by psychosocial indications and overrepresentation of disadvantaged families.

Subjects: the actual sample

The number of subjects that contributed to the analysis was 64. Nine cases were excluded for reasons noted in Table 3.1. Of the 97 families that were approached, 16 cases were involved only in the pilot study and 8 families refused to participate. The most frequent reasons were lack of time and apprehension at appearing before the videocamera.

Of the 64 families included in the main sample a number do not conform to all four of the population criteria mentioned above. One subject was two months past the age range; one was a month too young. Three cases with femur fractures were included although they did not experience surgery with full aneasthesia. One case of meningitis was included, although, of course, no surgery was indicated. The patients were expected to stay for a week but nine were discharged earlier. Six of them, with a duration of 5 or 6 days in hospital were retained; the other three were excluded from the analysis.

It was intended to include emergency admissions in the sample, in spite of the fact that data on prehospital adjustment are limited if a prehospital visit, in the home environment, is impossible. However, the recruitment procedures did not provide sufficient opportunity to contact more than six of these cases. The majority of emergency admissions at this age do not involve surgery.

Although admissions for elective surgery are planned in the hospital, often the planning is rescheduled and the date of surgery is known only a few days in advance. For the research team these cases had to be treated as emergency admissions; which means that information on prehospital adjustment is limited to questionnaires for nine cases.

TABLE 3.1   *Number of patients and their families*

Pilot study *)	sample size minus refusals and exclusions		$N = 16$
Main study	sample size minus refusals and exclusions		$N = 64$
	exclusions:	severe mental handicap	3	
		participation discontinued	2	
		death of child-patient	1	
		less than 5 days in hospital	3	
	total of exclusions:			9
	refusals			8

*) The pilot study is reported separately (Fahrenfort, Jacobs & Kaptein- de Kock van Leeuwen, 1990).

3.3   Design and assessments

Procedure

Before the first visit at home the families were assigned either to the experimental, or to the control group. Those in the experimental group received interventions. Interventions consisted of a booklet and consultation; both will be described in Section 3.4. Assignment was done purely at random for the first five cases. Afterwards a newly identified family was nearly always assigned to the experimental group if the consultant had the opportunity to arrange the consultation. For truly planned admissions, where cooperation was obtained at least one week in advance, the assignment therefore depended mainly on the question whether the consultant had new cases on hand or not, and therefore on the order of entry. The procedure was intended to achieve an effect similar to random assignment.

49

The first families that received interventions were treated with extra caution because the consultant had not yet tested her approach. She urged that these interventions should be classified as 'tentative' and not used to test the efficacy of the procedure. At the time of completion the sample contained:

    35 controls

    4 tentative interventions

    25 true interventions

Families were visited at home for prehospital assessments. This involved some exchange of general information, play sessions, recorded on videotape, and completion of several questionnaires. In the case of an emergency admission, or an admission that was fixed only at the last possible moment, the first contacts were planned in the hospital: nine cases. In two cases the hospital was the setting for the consultation. Normally, the probability of being assigned to interventions was nearly one half, but for emergency admissions it turned out to be only two out of nine, which reflects some bias. The effect of this is discussed in Section 7.1.

The family was subsequently visited in the hospital. A video record was obtained before surgery, except in three cases, where no opportunity was found to conduct the session before the operation was due. Data were collected concerning parental presence and participation in the hospital. After discharge the research team remained in touch with the parents. By telephone the posthospital behavior questionnaire was administered one month afterwards. Two months after discharge the complete posthospital assessment was conducted, by exactly the same standards as prehospital assessment. A final long-term follow up was scheduled to assess language development and possible long-term behavioral disturbances. As far as possible the time of follow-up was chosen at least nine months after discharge and not until the infant was two and a half years old.

The main body of data, excluding the late follow up, was collected by two investigators who had to establish rapport and make appointments with their own 'case load' of parents. Prehospital and posthospital assessment of one family was always performed by the same investigator. The extensive contacts required for appointments, explanations and data collection may have influenced parents. Parents from control-group-families rarely asked for advice, but may have been alerted to the problems of hospitalization by data collecting procedures.

Methodologically, blind assessment was clearly to be preferred, but it was impossible for the investigators to remain blind to interventions. The late follow-up was shared by all members of the research team. Sixty percent of the cases was done, however, by a graduate student who could not distinguish experimentals and controls.

Instruments: Questionnaires and tests

The *Background Questionnaire* is not a standardized instrument, but designed for the present investigation to obtain information on the family, the history of separation episodes experienced by the child, the medical history, and parental involvement in previous hospitalizations. It was administered in prehospital assessment.

The *Behaviour Screening Questionnaire (BSQ)* served to record behavioral disturbances. It is designed as a semi-structured interview with the parent by Richman, Stevenson and Graham (1982) in England. The twelve areas of behavior covered are: sleeping, eating, bowel control, attention seeking and dependency, relationships with other children, activity, concentration, ease of control, tempers, moods, worries and fears. The validity of the instrument was found to be satisfactory (Richman et al., 1982; Richman & Graham, 1971; Earls, Jacobs, Goldfein, & Silbert, 1982) in the Netherlands by Swets-Gronert (1986). Added to the basic list were a number of items concerning developmental landmarks and (psycho-)somatic complaints as conceived by Swets-Gronert. The BSQ was applied in prehospital and posthospital assessment as well as in the late follow up.

The *Parental Participation Questionnaire* is (newly) designed to record: caretaking of either parent (father and/or mother) in the hospital setting, presence during possibly stressful moments of nursing or diagnostic procedures, presence during the day, rooming-in, and presence at anaesthesia induction. It was obtained in interview fashion, during and after the sojourn in hospital.

The *Posthospital Behavior Questionnaire (PHBQ)*, an inventory specifically developed to record behavioral signs of upset and psychological improvement after hospitalization, was applied one month after discharge. The original design by Vernon and associates (Vernon & Schulman, 1964; Vernon, Schulman & Foley, 1966) was recently translated into Dutch and applied by Kaptein-de Kock van Leeuwen (1987). The instrument has been used in many studies. Its validity is amply confirmed and it has been found suitable for administration by telephone, as done in the present study (Davenport & Werry, 1970).

The *Nijmegen-California Kinder Sorteertechniek (NCKS)*, a Dutch version of the California Child Q-set (CCQ), developed in Nijmegen, is a Q-sort instructing the parents to judge the child on a hundred behavioral characteristics. The validity is documented to be quite satisfactory (Van Lieshout, Riksen-Walraven, Ten Brink et al., 1986). Among the traits that can be measured 'Ego-resilience' is a particularly useful index for socio-emotional adaptation. Ego-resilience refers to a general and widely relevant personal characteristic: flexibility and persistence in problem solving, exhibited in various situations. The concept has acquired a proven construct validity. The Q-set was employed in the late follow up.

The *Reynell Developmental Language Scales* (Reynell & Huntley, 1977) reflect understanding of spoken words and sentences as well as development of language production. The diagnostic power is slight in the second, but better in the third year of life. It was employed in the late follow up.

Instruments: Video episodes and ratings

Sensitivity dimensions of parental support could be rated from video-records taken at the patient's home. This allowed separate pre- and posthospital assessment. The recordings in the hospital have been used for different purposes, discussed below. Parental support and a valid rating system have been specified by Erickson, Sroufe and Egeland (1985) for the developmental stage considered in our study. In this procedure instructional assignments of a playful kind are given: activities that generate a mild tension, because they are not easy. The format is fifteen minutes of parent-child interaction, consisting of three separate 5-minute episodes. For every episode challenging instructional toys or games are provided with two grades of difficultness: 12-24 months and 25-36 months tasks. These episodes are preceded by fifteen minutes of free play, sufficient to overcome sensitivity to the camera and other artificial circumstances.

In video sessions at home only one parent is allowed to participate, in some cases the father (if he could be considered as a principal caretaker), more often the mother. Presence of other family members, including siblings is avoided. Participation is not allowed for them, except in the case of a twinbrother or -sister, which occured three times.

Three ratings, reflecting separate dimensions of parental support according to Erickson et al. (1985) were given for each 15-minute session:

Supportive Presence. This scale reflects the degree of support and encouragement offered by the parent, the reinforcement of confidence by parallel verbal and nonverbal cues.

Respect for Autonomy. This scale reflects the degree to which the parent recognizes and respects the child's individuality, motives and perspectives in the session.

Structure and Limit Setting. This scale reflects how adequately the parent attempts to establish his/her expectations of the child's behavior versus not communicating or not enforcing his/her agenda adequately.

Quality of Affective Sharing. This fourth rating employed a different (three point) rating scale as devised by Waters, Wippman and Sroufe (1979). The scale reflects qualitative aspects of affective and verbal exchanges, the child's initiative in the interactions, and the interest and enthusiasm shown in exchanges with the parent.

The four scales were combined to represent the concept *sensitivity.*

Disturbance of the relationship. While the first three ratings were concerned with behavior of the parents during interaction, and the fourth with the interaction itself, two additional ratings, produced by a different observer, were more concerned with behavior of the child during interaction:

Avoidance of the parent. This scale reflects the child's tendencies or clear attempts to avoid interacting with the parent.

Child negativity. Degree to which the child shows anger, dislike or hostility toward the parent. The two scales were combined during analysis to measure the concept disturbed relationship.

Attachment Quality was derived from video records in the hospital, bearing a degree of resemblance to the Strange Situation described in Section 1.3. The feasibility of this assessment was discussed and endorsed by three national experts in attachment research and Strange Situation Behavior, who first participated in a pilot experiment and later on contributed final Attachment Quality classifications.

A video session in the hospital was usually organized on the first or second day of hospital admission, before surgery. In contrast to the procedure in the home situation, no special activities were programmed, but a separation between child and parent(s) was scheduled at the start of the session. This was contrived in either one of two different arrangements. At the outset it was preferred to take advantage of "natural" separations, occurring at night or in the afternoon when the infant was supposed to sleep. A video-recorded reunion of infant and parent was, in this arrangement, planned in the early morning, or right at the end of the afternoon nap. If he was actually sleeping, the infant had to be awakened by the researcher first. Next he was filmed for five minutes without relatives present. The other arrangement required an "artificial" separation of ten minutes, which appeared to be more expedient in most circumstances. For both arrangements the parent(s) was (were) instructed to enter (consecutively) at an appointed moment, or if the infant was so distressed that he did not stop crying. In any case care was taken to record interaction at the time of reunion, in order to obtain a record that might be comparable to a Strange-Situation-reunion. Subsequent parent-child interaction was filmed contiguously for fifteen minutes. The parents were instructed to follow their ordinary course of caretaking or any other activity chosen. Although video-episodes in the hospital offer a more realistic picture of ordinary behavior than Strange Situation records, the variability of conditions is considerably larger. In spite of this lack of standard conditons, attempts to judge attachment qualities yielded encouraging results, judged by degree of consensus, reported in Chapter 4 (p. 70).

FIGURE 3.2 *The study design: General concepts measured and specific measurements, represented on an adjusted time axis*

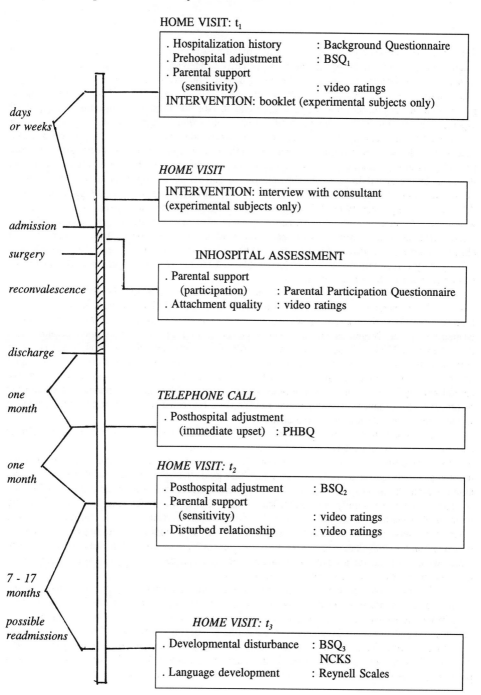

HOME VISIT: t_1

. Hospitalization history   : Background Questionnaire
. Prehospital adjustment   : BSQ_1
. Parental support
   (sensitivity)   : video ratings
INTERVENTION: booklet (experimental subjects only)

days or weeks

HOME VISIT

INTERVENTION: interview with consultant
(experimental subjects only)

admission

surgery

reconvalescence

INHOSPITAL ASSESSMENT

. Parental support
   (participation)   : Parental Participation Questionnaire
. Attachment quality   : video ratings

discharge

one month

TELEPHONE CALL

. Posthospital adjustment
   (immediate upset)   : PHBQ

one month

HOME VISIT: t_2

. Posthospital adjustment   : BSQ_2
. Parental support
   (sensitivity)   : video ratings
. Disturbed relationship   : video ratings

7 - 17 months

possible readmissions

HOME VISIT: t_3

. Developmental disturbance   : BSQ_3
                                NCKS
. Language development   : Reynell Scales

3.4   Interventions

Design of interventions

The goal of interventions, enhancement of the adequacy of parental support during hospitalization of the infant or toddler, was primarily conceived in terms of parental involvement as discussed in Section 1.2: attention should be paid to presence of parents in the daytime and at night, and a specific subject should be presence during induction of anaesthesia. During preparation of the program this scope was extended. Not just presence, but attitude and general aspects of interaction with, and support of, infants and toddlers might be important. On the other hand, practical limitations precluded extensive contacts with the consultant, therefore not much guidance could be offered during the actual hospitalization episode. It was decided to opt for a limited program, consisting of an instructional booklet and one visit by a 'consultant' to discuss the forthcoming hospitalization and the role of the parents. The hospital staff was not involved in this program. Enlistment of their support in six different hospitals would have been very difficult and the possibility of staff-members being able to distinguish experimental and control-group subjects seemed clearly undesirable. The person of the 'consultant' was carefully chosen. The consultant was a woman who had ample experience as pedagogical co-worker in a children's hospital, (incidentally one of the hospitals involved in the research project), and subsequently had acquired her degree. Her status as a mother of two children was considered an additional asset in the role of consultant.

The booklet that was used in the intervention-program was specifically written to offer basic advice to parents in the case of hospitalization of one of their children. It was called 'Je kind in het ziekenhuis; wat kun je als ouder doen?'['Children in hospital, options for parents'], written by M. van Bergen en M. van Gaalen, published in 1986 by Kosmos in cooperation with the national association 'Kind en Ziekenhuis'. Although it was intended for a wide age-range of childpatients and included some sections on verbal preparation (for older children) it was judged by the research team to be suitable for the present purpose, in view of its size (45 pages), careful approach and wording. This booklet was offered to every experimental family at the time of prehospital assessment. The mother or parents were requested to read it and comment upon it when visited, some days later, by the consultant.

It was anticipated that important differences would be found among families in their patterns of parent-child interaction and their views and intentions regarding participation in the hospital. Therefore it was decided to tailor the contents of the intervention interview to each individual family as far as possible. To attain this goal, the visit of the consultant was always planned after the prehospital assessment visit. This design permitted the consultant to become acquainted with the family and specifically with the child. Video-records obtained during prehospital assessment were viewed and discussed by the investigator and consultant together before the intervention visit. In this session a plan with some more specific objectives could be prepared for the consultation. Nevertheless, the general framework and a checklist of relevant topics were the same for all experimental families. The approach in terms of standardization of the contents of the interviews will be discussed below.

One of the viewpoints of the research-team is that the equal responsibility of father and mother should be acknowledged and occasionally emphasized. In spite of this basic principle it was frequently decided to arrange intervention interviews with one parent (the mother) alone if this was what she wished. This approach permitted a more personal contact and more openness regarding worries, fears, attitudes and intentions than an interview where three people were involved. Nevertheless the preference of the parents was accepted as decisive: ten times both parents, eighteen times only the mother and one time only the father were present at the intervention visit. Previous attempts to encourage parental attendance in hospital by Roskies (1979) have shown that efforts directed towards the mother increased paternal involvement appreciably.

Purport and standardization; specific topics

The research team, including the consultant, felt justifiably reluctant to urge parents toward attendance in the hospital without respect for their attitudes. Couture (1976) who, in his research on the effects of rooming-in, tried to establish a rooming-in and a control group on the basis of assignment, was forced to abandon his design because parents were not prepared to accept this interference. In the present study an attempt was made to help parents decide consciously, after appropriate information had been provided.

The booklet provided basic information as well as a point of departure for the interview. As far as the consultant could ascertain all mothers and fathers present had read the booklet, or at least some of it. The principal message: to be present as far as was possible and reasonable, was identified by many, but not all parents and could, if necessary, be reemphasized. Furthermore evaluative statements concerning the text were gathered, in order to be transmitted to the authors and the association 'Kind en Ziekenhuis'. The interview was conducted in an atmosphere of thinking along with the parents. The problems or questions generated from their viewpoint were discussed. The contents of the interview were moreover standardized by a checklist of relevant topics, composed at the outset of the project. This checklist contained the following subjects:
- presence during daytime;
- presence during induction of anaesthesia and aggravating treatment;
- rooming-in;
- the importance of a good understanding between parents and nurses, an assertive attitude on the part of the parent: asking questions and taking initiatives when necessary;
- father's share in presence and support, the possibility for him to be free of regular duties (frequently fathers undertook rooming-in);
- the possible stress of the coming events for siblings and the provisions for their care.
In addition the question was discussed whether any preparation of the child-patient was possible. Frequently it was suggested to obtain a set of toys mimicking a doctor's attributes.

A general principle was reinforcement of the parent's confidence where possible. Apprehension of parents relating to the forthcoming surgery was given due attention. The importance of honest communication toward the child, especially relating to presence and departure in the hospital was emphasized.

Finally, whenever appropriate, attention was given to conspicuous aspects of mother-child-interaction. The mother was encouraged to detect infant's or toddler's signals and respond accordingly wherever this kind of advice seemed to be useful. A more complete account of the interventions and the reasons behind several choices made in implementation is provided by Kaptein-de Kock van Leeuwen and Jacobs (1992).

3.5   Summing up

A research project has been presented in which various aspects of child-caregiver interactions are covered as well as possible, before, during and after hospitalization of the child. Parental support in hospital is the central theme. The attempt to promote parental participation can be evaluated by means of an experimental design. The last follow-up is scheduled at a time that implies complete recovery from temporary upset. The dependent variables include parental report, observation of child-caregiver interactions and language development.

The next chapter will serve to describe the sample and the degree of parental participation in the hospital. Moreover, the many instruments and scales will be tested and improved by psychometric standards.

CHAPTER 4 PRELIMINARY ANALYSIS OF THE SAMPLE AND THE
INSTRUMENTS

The present chapter serves to describe the sample first. General properties, like age and gender distributions are given and a complete list of medical problems is presented in Section 4.1. The instrument for recording parental attendance in hospital and a description of the degree of parental presence that was observed in the sample are treated in Section 4.2. Other questionnaires: the BSQ and the PHBQ are examined for internal consistency in Section 4.3. Finally, in Section 4.4 the measures that are based on video-ratings are subjected to preliminary analysis: measurements of sensitivity, of attachment-quality and of disturbance of relationship at the time of posttest.

4.1   General characteristics and medical descriptions of the sample

General characteristics

The criteria for sample selection, like upper and lower boundaries for age and expected time in hospital, have already been described. The background characteristics, medical history, the parental presence in hospital and behavioral problems in the sample will now be reviewed. Attention will be paid to pretest differences between the two groups of the design.

In the following description of the sample the 'tentative interventions' and 'true interventions', distinguished in Section 3.3, will be summarized into the category of 'interventions'; otherwise the manifold tables would be unnecessarily complex. The distinction will be heeded in the context of testing hypotheses, in Chapter 5.

The data on gender and age are to be found in Table 4.1. Boys make up the majority of the sample, 61%, and also of the population hospitalized at this age. The slightly different representation of the sexes within the groups of the design is of no consequence, since the sex

TABLE 4.1   *Gender and age at t_1: the time of pretest*

		whole sample	intervention group	control group
gender				
	male	39 (61%)	19	20
	female	25 (39%)	10	15
age at t_1				
	≤ 24 months	39 (61%)	18	21
	> 24 months	25 (39%)	11	14

difference is neutral to the independent variables and dependent variables studied here. Age, on the other hand, is relevant for outcome. The age distribution, displayed in Table 4.1, is nearly the same in the two groups; the mean is 22 months, the SD 8 in each case.

The number of siblings in the sample ranges from none to five. However, 42% of the patients has no siblings at all and another 40% just one, more often an older sister or brother. This is recorded here for the sake of description. The number of siblings is not related to the measures of adjustment, nor to the presence of parents in the hospital. This might have been different in a sample of older children with somewhat larger nuclear families.

In all families but one, both parents and the children lived together. One mother lived with her small daughter but without the father. Two more separations occurred during our investigations. One of the mothers involved initiated a new partnership before the long term follow-up.

The primary caretaker should also be the primary respondent, according to the design. Inquiry was made into the distribution of caretaking between parents. Usually the mother was the principal caretaker, but four couples claimed exactly equal shares and two fathers were designated primary caretakers and, therefore, respondents.

The ordinary involvement of fathers was roughly estimated by their participation in four types of caretaking behavior: playing with the child, changing diapers, feeding the child and bringing the child to bed. Eighty percent of the respondents reported some contribution of the father to each of the four activities. Only one father 'failed' all four, while the remaining fathers were in between.

Timing of the late follow-up

In the course of data collection it proved to be impossible to maintain fixed rules for the timing of the late follow-up. Two principles were followed: (1) to postpone the late follow-up till nine months past discharge from hospital, seven months after the posttest; (2) to postpone until children had reached an age of 24 months at least, preferably 30 months, because the instruments were less suitable for younger children. However, the pressure of time and other organizational circumstances necessitated departures from those rules. The effect of the policy was that the age at t_3 was more homogeneous than at t_1 and t_2. The mean time between discharge and late follow-up was one year. This distribution is shown in Table 4.2.

TABLE 4.2   *Timing of the late follow-up*

time between discharge and late follow-up	frequency	age at the time of late follow-up	frequency
6-7 months	1	22-25 months	8
8-9 months	14	26-29 months	8
10-11 months	19	30-33 months	19
12-13 months	9	34-37 months	7
14-15 months	9	38-41 months	8
16-17 months	6	42-45 months	7
18-19 months	3	46-49 months	4
20 months	1	50-53 months	1
M = 12 months	*SD* = 3 months	*M* = 34 months	*SD* = 7 months

The majority of patients already had a *history* of hospitalization. The history of their medical problems has been traced to the beginnings. Problems during pregnancy were mentioned by 20% of the mothers (parents). Delivery was more than two weeks early for 25%. Parturition was experienced to be particularly difficult by 32% of the sample. In 49% some defect of the newborn was established shortly after birth.

One important independent variable in the study is the previous hospitalization experience of the infants and toddlers. According to our hypothesis (2) preadmission adjustment and emotional vulnerability will be modified by previous hospitalizations. The sample is particularly suitable for investigating this hypothesis. Frequency of previous admissions is displayed in Table 4.3. It is evident that the effect of the prospectively studied admissions should be considered within the context of hospitalization history.

TABLE 4.3   *Frequency of previous admissions not counting one-day-admissions*

previous admissions	full sample	intervention group	control group
none	17 (27%)	7	10
1	22 (34%)	9	13
2	12 (19%)	6	6
3	5 (8%)	4	1
4	3 (5%)	1	2
5	3 (5%)	1	2
6	2 (3%)	1	1
total	64 (100%)	29	35
means	1.6	1.6	1.5

The experimental group is slightly at a disadvantage for previous admissions, but not if diagnostic categories are compared. The principal diagnoses in the sample are presented in Table 4.4.

As intended, a wide variety of medical problems is included. From a medical point of view, the domain of planned surgery at this developmental stage is adequately (although not completely) covered in the sample. Neurological surgery was not included, to avoid confounding problems. Oncological cases were not accessible and moreover might have presented serious problems for the researchers. Other diagnoses with considerable risk of mortality are included, primarily cases of heart surgery. Most of the problems pertain to congenital malformation, sometimes requiring diagnostic efforts and concomitant hospitalization. For a diagnosis like *congenital luxation of hips* or *anus atresia* a program of corrective measures or surgical interventions is standard; multiple hospitalizations are inevitable. In other cases previous admissions have occurred for a variety of reasons, not necessarily connected with the present diagnosis. The stress caused by a particular anomaly is partly dependent on the number of admissions required, partly on the additional impediments of normal behavior and development,

TABLE 4.4   *Frequency of diagnoses*

category	diagnosis		frequency
(1)	hypospadia		17
(2)	congenital gastro-intestinal disorders:		
	- diaphragmatic hernia with oesophagal reflux	5	
	- anus atresia	3	
	- Hirschsprung's disease	3	
	- congenital malformation of the gut (unspecified)	2	
	- congenital malformation of the gut (separated siamese twin)	1	
	- prune-belly	1	
	- volvulus	1	
	- webbing of the gut	1	
	subtotal:		17
(3)	congenital heart diseases:		
	- atrium septum defect II	6	
	- tetralogy of Fallot	4	
	subtotal:		10
(4)	cleft lip and palate		5
(5)	vesico-ureteral reflux		4
(6)	congenital luxation of hips		4
(7)	complicated femur fracture		3
(8)	mastoiditis		2
(9)	clubfoot		1
(10)	meningitis		1

for instance a stoma, immobilization or applications of plaster. A comparison of the experimental and control group in terms of diagnoses is made in Table 4.5.

TABLE 4.5   *Comparison of experimental and control group by diagnostic category*

	whole sample	interventions	controls
(1) hypospadia	17	9	8
(2) gastro-intestinal problems	17	9	8
(3) congenital heart disease	10	4	6
(4) cleft lip and palate	5	2	3
(5) vesico-ureteral reflux	4	0	4
(6) congenital luxation of hips	4	3	1
(7) miscellaneous	7	2	5

The distribution of cases among hospitals is shown in Table 4.6. This is only relevant for a comparison among the design groups. Undoubtedly differences among hospitals will affect the adjustment of patients and their families, but it was decided not to pursue such differences, because they will be confounded with the type of surgery.

TABLE 4.6   *Distribution among hospitals*

hospital	sample	interventions	controls
AZL (Leiden)	18	9	9
Clara hospital (Rotterdam)	2		2
JKZ (Den Haag)	12	5	7
R. de Graaf (Delft)	3		3
SKZ (Rotterdam)	18	10	8
AZ-VU (Amsterdam)	11	5	6
total	64	29	35

The sample is fairly evenly divided but for the fact that two hospitals are not represented in the experimental group, a possible cause of bias considered in Section 7.1. Geographically the sample is widely dispersed, with families living in forty-six different towns and villages.

The duration of admissions between pretest and posttest ranges from 5 to 25 days. An account of this factor in the two design groups is provided by Table 4.7. Intervention and control group are substantially the same here.

TABLE 4.7   *Duration of admissions between pretest and posttest*

duration category		sample	intervention	control
(1)	5-7 days	13	5	8
(2)	8-9 days	16	8	8
(3)	10-11 days	14	7	7
(4)	12-15 days	11	5	6
(5)	16-25 days	10	4	6
total		64	29	35

4.2   Scaling and observed distributions of parental attendance in hospital

A scale for parental participation in hospital

Parental support was distinguished into (a general factor of) sensitivity on the one hand and parental attendance or presence during the hospital treatment on the other. These aspects are positively correlated; in fact strongly: 0.59 ($p < .001$). This correlation is all the more remark-

61

able, because sensitivity has been measured at home, with methods that are completely unbiased in relation to the assessment of support in hospital. The finding suggests that both aspects of parental behavior are stimulated by recognition of the toddler's needs.

Parental presence in hospital was measured with a short questionnaire of nine items, as displayed in Table 4.8. Although presence in the daytime was recorded as presence of any parent or both parents, separate inclusion of the father's share in parental support and the practice of alternate caretaking seemed to be justified, as it reflects the attitude and cooperation of parents in the situation.

The scale was evaluated according to Cronbach's internal consistency procedure. Corrected r(i) is reported in Table 4.8; the figures are substantially positive or even high for all items.

TABLE 4.8   *Parental Participation Questionnaire: corrected item-total correlations*

		r(i)
(1)	Presence in the morning	.71
(2)	Presence in the afternoon	.62
(3)	Presence in the evening	.59
(4)	Presence during examinations etc.	.63
(5)	Presence at induction of anaesthesia	.45
(6)	Any rooming-in	.58
(7)	Rooming-in proportional to duration	.58
(8)	Father's involvement	.50
(9)	Alternate caretaking	.46

The weight that should be given to any aspect of parental involvement is somewhat arbitrary. For example: it is not known whether rooming-in for a few nights only, as recommended in some hospitals, is nearly as beneficial as consistent rooming-in, nor whether rooming-in is more or less important than presence in the daytime. The number of nights spent by parents who practice rooming-in is not a good measure because it may be related to duration of hospitalization, therefore the proportion of nights is a better measure. Anyhow, standard deviations of items do not reflect their support value. One step in giving a presumably sensible weight to rooming-in was the separate inclusion of a dichotomous score (of zero or one) for any rooming-in and a score for the proportion of nights. Even so, considering standard deviations of these rooming-in items, their unweighted contribution is too small in comparison to other items. Since artificial weighing is arbitrary in any case, it was decided to give equal weight to any of the items presented here. This end is achieved by standardization of all itemscores: they were transformed to z-scores. By this transformation internal consistency was slightly increased: coefficient alpha was .82 before standardization and .85 afterwards. From a psychometric viewpoint the final scale is very satisfactory.

Degree of parental presence in hospital

The parental participation in the sample, both in the control- and experimental group, was *high* compared to expectations based on the literature (cited in 1.2) and on our earlier retrospective study described in Chapter 2. Both standards for comparison reflect the practices that were common in 1986.

Because the degree of parental involvement and its influence on the child is our main theme, a quantitative account of parental activity is indispensable. Unfortunately an evocative, literary, description of events in hospital is not in line with the demands of a scientific account, although it might be useful for an understanding of the process and the strain on parents and patients. Frequently, though not always the private needs of parents seemed to be forgotten during days and nights of caretaking or just 'being there'. Naturally the emotional burden for parents depends on many circumstances other than time spent in hospital: the condition of the child, the social atmosphere of the ward, etcetera.

Some parents meet the challenge by always operating as a couple: they are together in the hospital or not at all. In other families the primary responsibility seems to lie with the mother; the contribution of the father is limited to visits after working hours. In three cases the father was the primary caretaker in the hospital. The presumably most effective practice of

TABLE 4.9   *Presence in the hospital at daytime: frequencies for each daily period*

	mornings	afternoons	evenings
not present	2	-	2
0 to 1 hour	3	-	7
1 to 2 hours	4	3	14
2 to 3 hours	11	10	41
3 to 4 hours	44	51	-[1]
total	64	64	64

alternate caretaking, for parts of the day and/or for spending the night, was chosen by 21 couples: nearly one third of the sample.

The hours spent in hospital were recorded as accurately as possible, but this presented difficulties if no fixed schedule applied. The day of surgery was nearly always different, as was the day of admission and of discharge. Of course other shifts occurred. In final coding estimates were made of the average number of hours spent in hospital in the morning, the afternoon and the evening. Presence was counted if one parent or both parents were present, disregarding other relatives or visitors. The final distribution is presented in Table 4.9.

Rooming-in was possible in all of the participating hospital-wards. The only restriction was made in the SKZ where rooming-in was (is) officially not allowed for more than three nights, except in special circumstances. (Actually 5 cases out of 18 were allowed more than three nights.) The number of nights spent by parents with their child in hospital is sometimes impressive, as testified by Table 4.10. Table 4.11 provides further information on rooming-in.

---

[1]   The count for presence in the evening involved a maximum of three hours, in order to avoid confusion with rooming-in.

TABLE 4.10   *Frequency of rooming-in and persistence of parents in this practice*

number of nights	sample frequency	number of nights	sample frequency
0	23	7	2
1	5	8	5
2	5	9	3
3	2	10	2
4	3	11	2
5	7	14	1
6	2	18	2

An important feature of parents' participation is their presence at induction of anaesthesia. Fortunately most of the parents have been offered the opportunity to attend, and actually have been present. Unfortunately, this outcome is different from what might have been expected in many other hospitals (cf. Section 1.2) and precludes an analysis of the effects of this policy. The state of affairs is seen in Table 4.11.

TABLE 4.11   *Rooming-in related to length of admission (a) and presence at induction of anaesthesia (b)*

choice (a)	sample frequency	*	choice (b)	sample frequency
no rooming-in	23	*	absent at induction	5
partial rooming-in	21	*	present at induction	55
consistent rooming-in	20	*	no anaesthesia	4

4.3   Questionnaires: preliminary analysis

The Behaviour Screening Questionnaire (BSQ)

The BSQ is designed to detect behavior difficulties of children at preschool age from a structured interview with parents. It also covers various aspects of health, development and physical handicaps, but some of these subjects are not included in our analysis and will therefore be ignored in the present discussion. The problem-behavior scale is our principal criterion for general socio-emotional adjustment.

Twelve behavioral domains are selected by the original authors to construct the scale of problem behavior; two additional behavioral domains covered in the questionnaire are not included in this scale. To avoid confusion we will not refer to these behavioral domains as 'items' (as done by Richman & Graham, 1971) but as 'topics'. Every topic is scored according to one or more items (single questions) in the questionnaire as can be seen from Table 4.12.

64

TABLE 4.12   *Topics and items of the BSQ*

behavioral problem scale:		
topic (1)	eating problem	3 items
topic (2)	sleeping problem	3 items
topic (3)	soiling	3 items
topic (4)	hyperactivity	1 item
topic (5)	concentration	1 item
topic (6)	relationships	2 items
topic (7)	dependency	3 items
topic (8)	noncompliance	1 item
topic (9)	fits of anger	1 item
topic (10)	mood	1 item
topic (11)	worries	1 item
topic (12)	fears	12 items
additional scales:		
topic (13)	habits	8 items
topic (14)	somatic complaints	6 items

For every item a three point rating scale is employed as follows:
itemscore 0   problematic behavior absent
itemscore 1   problematic behavior present in mild degree not very frequent
itemscore 2   problematic behavior present in marked degree or frequent.
Both individual items and topics were rated by the authors along these three point rating scales. The inter-rater-reliability for scores on topics was calculated by the authors as a percentage of agreement; the range of outcomes was 57% to 100%. This criterion refers to separate scorings of the same taped interview. When separate interviews of the same case were compared agreement per topic fluctuated from 36% to 84%. The validity of each topic was judged by its potential to discriminate children attending a psychiatric clinic and a control group. Every topic of the scale could significantly discriminate these groups at the .05 level of significance, except (5) concentration, (9) tempers and (12) fears. The latter topics were maintained, as exclusion did not improve the discriminating power of the scale (Richman & Graham, 1971).

The stability of BSQ-scores was investigated by Swets Gronert (1986) on a sample of 60 unselected Dutch children, followed from the age of three to the age of five years. The Pearson correlation of total scores was .61 (p <.001) across a time span of two years, which indicated marked stability at this (early) developmental stage. Correlations on individual topics ranged from .20 to .53; this stability was significant (at .05 level, onesided) for all but two of these topics; the exceptions being (6) relationships: r = .20 and (7) dependency: r = .21. Altogether these results suggest considerable reliability for the total behavioral problem scale. The homogeneity of the scale, computed as alpha by Swets Gronert, was .66. This modest value should not surprise us, as scoring methods imply that scores for strongly related items are not entered separately in this computation, but are previously joined into scores for topics reflecting dissimilar behavioral domains.

The validity of the behavior problem scale as a criterion of behavioral development was firmly supported by the study of Swets-Gronert. In a multiple regression analysis BSQ problem-scores of five-year-olds could be 'predicted' linearly from temperament scores collected at the age of 2 and 3 years. In this equation the constructs: 'Difficult Temperament' and 'Unadaptable' served to explain 30% of criterion-variance at age five (adjusted for shrinkage). 43% (adjusted) could be explained by adding BSQ-scores collected at the age of three.

A factor analysis on the 12 topics of the behavior problem scale reported by Swets-

Gronert, yielded a distinction of externalizing and internalizing behavior difficulties. These two factors, however, left two thirds of the total variance unaccounted for. For this reason the separate analysis for these types of behavior will not be pursued here.

In reconstructing the behavioral problem scale for the present sample our predilections should be reviewed. As far as possible it is useful to replicate the original scale. Unfortunately two of the main topics, to be discussed below, are not appropriate for the age range 12-36 months, the range of our population. This is a serious drawback when the scale is used to discriminate 'normal' children from those who attend psychiatric clinics or are in need of similar treatment. Much of the discussion of Richman & Graham (1971), Earls, Jacobs, Goldfein, Silbert, Beardslee & Rivinus (1982), Richman et al. (1982) and Swets Gronert (1986) concerns the choice of cutting scores and the validity of the ensuing dichotomy. This issue need not concern us, as the principal purpose of our study is to clarify the relationship between BSQ-scores and predictors, such as hospitalization history and parental support. Therefore we are mainly interested in the behavioral content and relevance of topics and in the psychometric properties of the scale. Most of the topics mentioned in Table 4.12 have been implicated as symptoms of posthospital disturbance, as testified by their inclusion in the PHBQ (see Table 4.13).

The composition and scoring for the BSQ adopted here should be justified by examining the list of topics and the specific items involved. For this purpose due attention will be paid to the corrected item total correlation $r(i)$. Correlations of items with the remainder were computed with the help of a provisional scale with all 14 topics added.

(1) *eating problem*. This topic involves three items:

> b1   : poor appetite
> b2   : faddiness about food
> b3   : eating of non-food (e.g. paper)

In the original scoring, preferred here, the topic was scored as a marked problem if any of the items was scored as such. Arithmetically the maximum of scores on one of these items was the one that counts. According to this rule the $r(i)$ for eating problem was .32. Computing a *sum* of the three items as a subscale resulted in a lower $r(i)$; therefore this alternative was dismissed. The score for *eating problem* can not be regarded as a subscale, except for exploratory purposes.

(2) *sleeping problem*. This topic involves three items:

> b21   : bedtime resistance $r(i) = .17$
> b22   : waking at night $r(i) = .28$
> b23   : sleeping in parents' bed $r(i) = .38$

The items refer to commonly observed posthospital disorders and require specific attention as symptoms of upset and problems for parents. As we wanted to give sleeping problems a proper weight, and retain the itemscores in later analysis, all three were entered into the total problemscore. Although the three items are intercorrelated positively, a subscale constructed from them is too short to be regarded as a separate criterion, except for exploratory purposes.

(3) *soiling*. For the majority in our sample toilet training had not been completed, or not even started. Therefore items relating to this topic reflect a stage of development and can not be a measure of behavioral disturbance in our study.

(4,5) *hyperactivity / concentration problem*. These topics each belonged to the original score for behavior difficulties. $r(i)$ for hyperactivity is .28 and for concentration problems .16. Both behavioral problems may reflect posthospital disturbance. These single-item-topics were each included in the same fashion as in the original scale.

(6) *relationships*. This topic involves two items:

> b43   : relationships with siblings $r(i) = -.10$

b44   : relationships with peers $r(i) = +.34$

Like most of the original items both may reflect posthospital disturbance. The item-total-correlation for b43 was disappointing and sheds some doubt on the validity. We attribute this failure to the difference in developmental stage between patients and their siblings. Even the correlation between b43 and b44 is only +.07. After reflection it was decided to score 'relationships' just according to b44, and discard b43.

(7)   *dependency*. The items are:

    b45   : attention seeking $r(i) = .46$
    b46   : separation protest $r(i) = .40$
    b47   : cannot be left with babysitter $r(i) = .20$

Like the items concerning sleep disturbances these are vital to the content of a scale for assessment of posthospital disturbance and should be analysed as separate topics.

(8,9)   *noncompliance / fits of anger*.

$r(i) = .49$ for topic (8) and .40 for topic (9). Both were included in the scale, according to the original design.

(10)   *moods*. $r(i)$ for this item/topic is .40. It was included as in the original design.

(11)   *worries*. This topic could not be scored validly in our sample of age 12-36 months. It was discarded.

(12)   *fears*. The domain of fears was scored with the help of 12 items referring to specific fears. For this particular topic Richman and Graham (1971) provide a scoring instruction:

Is somewhat afraid of 1 or 2 things or has no fears   0
Has 1 or 2 marked fears or 3-5 fears altogether   1
Has 3 or more marked fears or 6 or more fears altogether   2

Apparently the authors have not analysed the psychometric aspects of specific fears. Our analysis indicated that individual fears have different patterns of linear relationships with other variables. For example, while *fear of the dark* has a connection, both to other fears and to the total problem scale, fear of insects is related to neither. For this reason it was abolished, together with fear of *cats, dogs* and *escalators*. $r(i)$ for these items ranged from -.09 to +.16. The remaining fear-items had $r(i) = +.24$ to $r(i) = +.39$. When items were added, into a scale of fears, the alpha for this scale was .54. This is a modest figure; nevertheless the scale of fears may have some validity as a separate measure. Of course it should be remembered that the standard deviation of this small scale is four or five times as large as that of other topics, therefore rescaling was desirable in the definition of a total problem score. The score of fears was now computed according to the original instruction. This correlated .91 with the sum of fears. The $r(i)$ of the topic was the same, viz. +.48 so for rescaling the original instruction was maintained.

additional scales (not employed in the final analysis)

(13)   *habits*. 8 items were involved in this topic, that was *not* included in the behavior-screening score. Two of them were discarded for insufficient variance and ensuing low values for $r(i)$. One more was dismissed for negative $r(i)$. For the other five $r(i)$ was between +.13 and +.39. These are:

    b24   : head banging
    b26   : nervous movements, like blinking
    b27   : hairpulling etcetera
    b29   : sucking thumb or fingers
    b30   : sucking many objects.

Most habits are infrequent, which may for some part explain low correlations and a low alpha (.33) for this cluster.

(14)   *physical   complaints*. Six items are available concerning either purely somatic or

psychosomatic complaints:

b9   : vomiting attacks
b10   : stomach ache
b11   : headache
b13   : any pains
b18   : constipation
b19   : diarrhoea.

Unlike the other topics, the meaning of these complaints is somewhat ambiguous: purely somatic or psychosomatic problems may be involved. Since alpha was only .15 this is not a useful scale according to our standards.

Reconstruction of the scale. In this revision of the scale, small departures from the original have been justified for the sake of psychometric improvement. As to item-content the original scale was maintained with two exceptions. Excluding *soiling* and *worries* left us with ten topics out of the original twelve. Alpha was computed for the composite. Reliability analysis reveals r(i) values for the problemscale items between +.16 and +.53. The homogeneity of the scale has been improved; alpha is now .70. Internal consistency is thus somewhat better than the .66 reported by Swets-Gronert (1986) for the original scale. Interrater reliability of the problem-behavior scale was examined by separate scoring of eight BSQ-interviews on tape. The agreement between scores of the two investigators was computed as a Pearson correlation, yielding .83 (p < .01).

The Post-Hospital Behavior Questionnaire (PHBQ)

The PHBQ was constructed by Vernon and his co-workers (Vernon & Schulman, 1964; Vernon, Schulman & Foley, 1966) to identify behavioral symptoms of upset in response to hospitalization. In support of the validity Vernon et al. (1966) reported a correlation of .47 between PHBQ scores and ratings of an independent interview with parents, conducted by a child psychiatrist. They reported a test-retest reliability of .65, as found by Cassell, who administered the instrument three days after hospitalization and again after one month. Their own findings, particularly the age related response patterns, confirm the validity of the questionnaire.

In the original version of Vernon et al. (1966) the PHBQ consisted of 27 items. It was designed for a broad age range. For our population, aged 12-36 months, nine items were deemed unsuitable. For the present investigation these were replaced by eight newly designed items, as specified in Table 4.13. To gauge the effect of this revision afterwards, provisional scales were computed for the original and the new items. The scale of original items correlated .51 (p < .01) with the sum of new items and .92 with total scores, so the choice of new items was confirmed.

The revised scale was tested by the standards of Cronbach's model for internal consistency; coefficient alpha was .74. Item 11: 'afraid of the dark' had to be discarded for zero variance. Three others had negative or zero correlations with the rest. Item 9: 'cannot be left with baby-sitter' proved to be inadequate because children were rarely or never left with a baby-sitter within the first weeks after hospitalization. Item 15: 'uninterested/apathetic' had insufficient variance and the same was true of item 24: 'change of habits' (unspecified). All in all, four items had to be discarded. A survey of all items is presented in Table 4.13.

68

TABLE 4.13 *Items, itemselection and corrected item-total correlations of the PHBQ*

items scored for improvement or deterioration	original items	new items	corrected r(i)	
1. resistance at bedtime	*		.39	
2. takes time to fall asleep	*		.34	
3. wakes up crying	*		.25	
4. sleeps with parents		*	.40	
5. lack of appetite	*		.26	
6. (other) eating problem	*		.43	
7. cannot be left alone for a while	*		.33	
8. follows mother in the home	*		.39	
9. cannot be left with baby-sitter		*	-.06	discarded
10. afraid or shy with stranger	*		.36	
11. afraid of the dark	*		-.00	discarded
12. afraid of doctors/hospital	*		.24	
13. more fearful		*	.13	
14. sometimes inaccessible	*		.32	
15. uninterested/apathetic	*		.02	discarded
16. does not amuse him/herself		*	.27	
17. frequently asks for help	*		.18	
18. fits of anger	*		.32	
19. breaks toys or objects	*		.31	
20. unmanageable	*		.28	
21. attention seeking	*		.57	
22. needs frequent cuddling		*	.24	
23. difficulties with playmates		*	.33	
24. change of habits	*		-.09	discarded
25. more demanding for parent		*	.26	
26. developmental progress		*	.34	

4.4 Video-ratings

Sensitivity measures

The fifteen-minute video episodes in pretest and posttest that constituted the raw material for assessment of sensitivity were described in Section 3.3, as were the sensitivity measures, originally developed by Erickson et al. (1985) and Waters et al. (1979). The ratings were assigned by two coders after elaborate training. In this procedure video-episodes that were difficult to interpret were discarded. In eleven cases no home video sessions in the pretest were available. 43 Cases of the pretest and 53 cases of the posttest could be scored. The inter-rater agreement was computed on eleven cases rated by both judges; the Pearson correlations are displayed in Table 4.14. This measure of reliability is high.

Each of the four dimensions has a distinct meaning and relevance, but for the purpose of measuring the construct 'sensitivity' they should be added. To investigate the assumption that the four are related to a common construct, intercorrelations were computed from the pretest. The highest correlation, .75 (p < .01), was found between *Respect for Autonomy* and *Supportive*

TABLE 4.14   *Pearson correlations for two independent judges of sensitivity; n = 11*

Supportive Presence	.94	(p <.01)
Respect for Autonomy	.96	(p <.01)
Structure and Limit Setting	.97	(p <.01)
Affective Sharing	.85	(p <.01)

Presence, the lowest .38 (p < .01), between *Respect for Autonomy* and *Structure and Limit Setting*. The posttest data gave similar results, therefore all scores can be considered as items of 'sensitivity'. When they were added the corrected item-total-correlation, r(i) ranged from .69 to .81 and coefficient alpha for this four item scale turned out to be .83; reflecting a high degree of internal consistency.

Because of the large number of missing values a comparison of pretest-posttest differences was useless. The two measurements were combined. The mean was taken when two observations were available.

Attachment Quality

The methods for rating attachment quality, based on the Strange Situation, were described in Section 1.3. In the present investigation, as explained in Section 3.3, video-records taken in the hospital served as material in the assessment of attachment quality. The feasibility of valid attachment classification on this material was first explored in an experiment. Classifications were produced by three experts in attachment-theory, trained thoroughly in rating Strange Situations. The fifteen-minute video-episodes in hospital wards used in this experiment were taken at random from the pilot study (four cases) and the sample (six cases). These cases were considered interchangeable for the purpose, because no change was made in the standards for a video-record in hospital after the pilot study. The only data available to the judges were the child's age and reason for hospitalization. Only the three principal categories (A, B & C) are considered in this experiment and in the subsequent analysis.

Five rating scales were employed to specify behavior at the time of reunion and afterwards:

I   Proximity- and contact-seeking behavior
II   Contact maintaining behavior
III   Resistant behavior
IV   Avoidant behavior
V   Affective sharing

Scales I to IV are standard scales for the analysis of Strange Situation behaviors; V is an extra scale designed by Waters et al. (1979) and is included here because it was thought helpful for final classification.

The results of the experiment are described in Table 4.15.

The inter-rater reliability was computed as the percentage of agreement between each pair of judges. The distinction secure attachment (B) versus insecure attachment (A or C) was considered the most important, therefore in this comparison agreement on security was calculated, yielding:
- agreement of judges I and II: 77%
- agreement of judges I and III: 77%
- agreement of judges II and III: 70%

TABLE 4.15   *Classification of attachment quality from videorecords in hospital by three expert judges; n = 10*

		attachment classification		
identification code		judge I	judge II	judge III
pilot cases	C2	B	B	B
	C1	C	A	A
	J3	B	B	B
	A1	B	B	B
sample cases	A2	B	B	B
	J6	B	A	B
	J7	A	A	B
	C3	-	B	A
	A11	B	A	A
	A18	B	B	B

Another indication of agreement was derived from the separate scales involved in the analysis. Pearson correlations were computed for each pair of judges. Findings are in Table 4.16.

From Table 4.16 it may be concluded that the percentage of agreement calculated between pairs of judges is not a chance result, even if coefficients are not very stable in this limited subsample. The negative correlation found for avoidance in one comparison is somewhat disconcerting. As it was decided to contrast securely attached and not-securely attached children the difference of A versus C will be of minor importance. Altogether the results suggest considerable agreement. There is no reason to exclude one of the judges. The findings were

TABLE 4.16   *Pearson correlations for separate scales in attachment classification; n = 10*
*   * is printed if p < .01*

	pairs of judges		
dimension	I II	I III	II III
proximity and contact seeking	.17	.64	.82*
contact maintenance	.90*	.65*	.98*
resistant behavior	.80*	.80*	.78*
avoidant behavior	.26	-.47	.43
affective sharing	.77*	.91*	.82*

interpreted to sustain the supposition that valid classification of attachment quality from video recordings in hospital is possible.

Subsequently every case was processed by one of the experts. Since video episodes could not be used in five of 64 cases (because of various practical obstacles) an attachment classification was obtained for 59 patients/families. The distribution of attachment qualities is displayed as Table 4.17.

TABLE 4.17   *Attachment classifications from hospital situations; N = 64*

attachment quality		frequency
Avoidant	Type A	18
Secure	Type B	37
Ambivalent	Type C	4
missing data		5

Disturbance of relationship

Two measures of child behavior that might indicate disturbance of the relationship were produced in the same way as the sensitivity ratings: *avoidance* and *negativity*. They were rated, according to the original instructions, provided by the author of the study in which they were developed (Erickson et al., 1985). Instructions for rating avoidance are reproduced as Appendix 2.1 , instructions for rating negativity are reproduced as Appendix 2.2. Materials for this rating procedure were the posttest videorecords of parent-child interaction during instructional tasks described in Section 3.3. The ratings were given by a observers unacquainted with sensitivity scores. They were only produced for mother-child interaction tasks during posttest sessions.

The inter-rater agreement was computed on a series of nine cases. It was .75 (p < .01) for avoidance and .71 (p < .05) for negativity. These values are low compared to the findings for sensitivity variables, but sufficient to have some faith in the rating procedure.

The correlation of avoidance and negativity was .80 (p < .01), which indicates that the two concepts tend to overlap. This is no objection to constructing a score for disturbance of relationship, by adding the two subscores.

4.5   Summing up

An analysis and description of the sample yields a variety of medical (surgical) problems, as has been intended. There are no reasons to question the representivity of the sample. Minor caveats concerning the comparison of experimentals and controls will be addressed in Section 7.1. Instruments and scales have been checked, in order to measure the following constructs:
  - hospitalization history
  - preadmission adjustment / behavior problems
  - parental sensitivity
  - initial attachment security
  - parental attendance in hospital
  - short-term upset after discharge
  - behavior problems (maladjustment) during follow-up
  - disturbance of relationship to caregiver
  - ego-resilience
  - language development

The method of analysis selected to test the hypotheses will be explained and applied in the next chapter.

CHAPTER 5 TESTING HYPOTHESES: DETERMINANTS OF POSTHOSPITAL ADJUSTMENT AND EFFECTS OF INTERVENTIONS

The purpose of this chapter is to present principal results, primarily results of testing the hypotheses formulated in Section 3.1. First the method of analysis will be explained. Hypotheses are tested with analysis of covariance as statistical tool. Section 5.2 will be devoted to a succinct review of constructs and variables, including a few correlations among them. In Section 5.3 the influence of previous hospitalizations is elucidated. In Section 5.4 the effect of experimental interventions will be evaluated. In Section 5.5 hypotheses are tested concerning effects of parental support and security of attachment on posthospital adjustment. In Section 5.6 language development will be related to the circumstances of hospitalization.

5.1   Purposes and tools of analysis

The goal of the analysis, and indeed of the whole research effort, is to unravel various influences on the adjustment of hospitalized children, such as previous hospitalization history, judicious consultation offered to parents, attachment quality and parental support. The effect of consultation is the only condition that can be tested by strictly experimental standards. To test the efficacy of the consultation program the experimental group of families will be compared to controls. Other conditions, for example hospitalization history and attachment quality could not be manipulated. Nevertheless these conditions require investigation for their possible impact. One of the problems in answering research questions of this second kind is the difference of *previous* conditions between groups that are selected to be different on a specific variable, for instance attachment quality. Because of the nonexperimental approach, only a modest degree of confidence is justified in an analysis that adjusts for previous differences (Cook & Campbell, 1979). Nevertheless it is this possibility that makes analysis of covariance, ANCOVA, the most attractive approach for the present data.

In applying ANCOVA a dependent variable is specified, while the sample is split into a number of categories (cells) according to one or more independent variables. The variance of the dependent variable is decomposed into variance between cell means, that may be related to the independent variable(s) and variance within cells, that serves as a standard to judge the significance of the former. The effects can be adjusted for preexisting differences, identified by covariates, representing influences unrelated to the causal factor to be tested. In testing experimental effects the introduction of covariates is useful because even in the case of random assignment preexisting differences may occur by chance. The method offers compensation for this inequality, whereas power is increased. When non-experimental effects are investigated, the need to control a number of conditions, either by introducing them as simultaneous independent variables or as covariates is even more urgent.

A disadvantage of the method is the necessity to enter independent variables as categories. To this end a continuous variable must be discreticized. The choice of categories or cutting points may be a difficult, or at times a rather arbitrary decision. A small number of levels (categories) implies loss of information and some concomitant loss of testing power. A large number of levels is not feasible for the present sample, because small or zero frequencies within cells may result. We preferred to distinguish only two levels and, with two exceptions described in the next section, to dichotomize variables near the mean in order to investigate their effects as independent variables.

The choice of covariates in various tests of hypotheses may be equally difficult. It was not considered wise to test a number of covariates for their correlations with each dependent variable and then make a selection, nor to enter a very large set of covariates, including any knowledge on previous history, regardless of significance. Three conditions, known at the time of pretest, appeared to be relevant, or in some analyses important: age, number of previous admissions longer than one day, and pretest adjustment as measured by the BSQ. These variables were selected as a standard set to correct ANOVA comparisons concerning the subsequent hospitalization and readjustment process. Even if these covariates make little difference, or act to reduce some important effect size, there seems to be no justification for omitting any one of them. In decomposing sums of squares these covariates were evaluated and partialled out first of all, next main effects were evaluated and, finally, first-order interactions. The number of independent variables in one analysis never exceeded two; this choice precluded empty cells and complexities of second order interactions. The test of some hypotheses is just the first-order interactional effect.

In order to report essential data of a large number of computations, tables were constructed without mean squares or sums of squares. On the other hand, cell means and standard deviations were considered essential for interpreting results. A choice had to be made between reporting means adjusted by covariates, or raw observed means. Although both may be relevant, the raw observed means are displayed. Of course the means will indicate whether an effect is in the expected direction; the F-value in itself gives no clue. In fact all hypotheses laid down in Section 2.1 are one-directional.

A one-sided test is performed when only effects in the predicted direction are considered significant. Therefore the critical region of the F-distribution, where one degree of freedom for the effect is available, should include any $p < .10$ in order to maintain alpha at .05. The p-value obtained for a specific test can be halved (in this situation) if effects are in the predicted direction. This correction was actually applied in Tables 5.2, 5.3 and 5.4, but not in other tables, because other tables contained one or more unexpected results. Because of one-sided testing, unexpected effects, (as found for example with security as independent in Table 5.9) are never significant.

Much thought was given to the choice between ANCOVA, with a single dependent variable, and MANCOVA (multivariate analysis of covariance) where a number of dependent variables are entered and tested simultaneously. MANCOVA is to be preferred where a number of related (correlated) dependent variables are available that have a similar theoretical status, for example a number of repeated measures. In our design one measurement is repeated (the BSQ), other outcome measures, like PHBQ, disturbed relationship and ego-resilience are, for various good reasons, not repeated, nor simultaneously measured. This heterogeneity of criterion measures will be discussed in the next section. As for power, Tabachnik and Fidell (1989) suggest that ANOVA should be preferred in many circumstances. Herzog and Rovine (1985) maintain that, in the case of repeated measures, ANOVA is more powerful than MANOVA; however, the assumptions are more restrictive. It was decided to opt for ANOVA, or rather ANCOVA, and check assumptions.

The critical (for hypothesis testing) variables have unimodal, roughly normal distributions. An exception is the distribution of *hospital days*, days spent in previous hospital episodes, which is rather skewed, as can be seen in Table 4.3 (p. 59). The distribution of disturbance of relationship was skewed as well. Transformations were not deemed necessary, however. To check for homogeneity of variances and covariances the tests of Cochran, Bartlett and Box were performed where appropriate. In a few cases Cochrans's C and the Bartlett-Box F turned out to be significant at the .05 level. In such cases no ANCOVA was performed, but rather a nonparametric test of difference like Mann-Whitney. Wherever F-tests are reported the tell-tale statistics are insignificant.

5.2.   Conceptual and empirical relations between variables

Before entering upon a description of results, particularly refutation or support of hypotheses, the 'cast' of variables must be reviewed. A distinction is made here between:
(a)   *preconditions:* variables referring to the time of pretest (t_1) or even earlier, mainly employed as covariates.
(b)   *process variables:* conditions during hospitalization (t_{1-2}) that are presumed to be influential to the outcome, mainly employed as independent variables in the analysis.
(c)   *posttest variables:* measures of upset or adjustment after hospitalization, at time t_2, mainly employed as dependent variables in the analysis.
(d)   *long-term follow-up:* measures of disturbance or adjustment, at least nine months after discharge: t_3 always employed as dependent variables.
The variables are summarized in Figure 5.1 (page 78). The four categories of variables will be briefly discussed.

(a)   *Preconditions*
Implications of age are emphasized in the theoretical review. Although no hypothesis is put forward about age-related differences within the selected span of 12 - 36 months, it was prudent to enter age as a covariate. Many age-related differences were observed.

Hospitalization history is indexed by two variables: number of previous admissions and cumulative number of previous hospital days. The first hypothesis, concerning their main effects on prehospital adjustment, was tested for each variable. Since the two measures correlate .75, it makes little sense to enter both as covariates. The number of previous admissions, a measure that can be produced in most circumstances, was post hoc selected to represent hospitalization history.

BSQ_1, the pretest BSQ, is within our design, the most valid operational definition of 'prehospital' (which means: previous to the *selected* hospital episode) adjustment. It serves as a covariate, firstly to correct the prediction of any ANCOVA, secondly because it is of specific relevance to enter a pretest BSQ-measure as covariate, when subsequent BSQ-measures are itended to reflect possible change. Where BSQ_1 serves as independent variable it is cut at the mean.

(b)   *Process variables*
The variables intervention and duration require no further comment.

Security of attachment is grouped here among the process variables. Because it is based - with three exceptions - on records taken only one, two or three days after admission, it is thought to represent the initial status, an independent variable that may modify the process. As an independent variable it is divided into three categories: secure, insecure and unknown (five cases are unknown, but must not be discarded). It might be conjectured that parental support and security should be linked in some way. This, however, is not true. Security correlates .07 with sensitivity and .04 with parental presence.

FIGURE 5.1   *Variables involved in hypotheses*

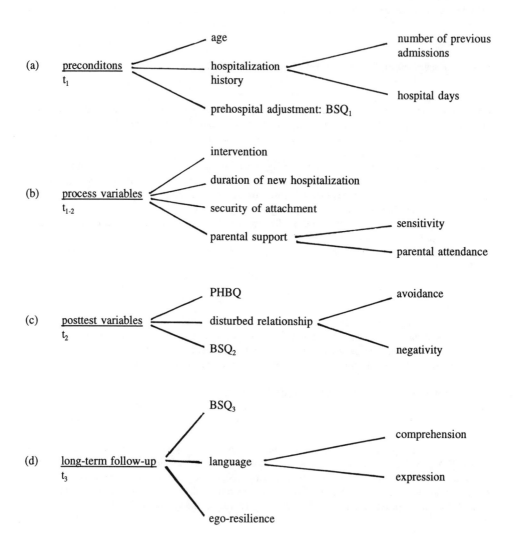

(a)   preconditons
      t_1
      - age
      - hospitalization history
        - number of previous admissions
        - hospital days
      - prehospital adjustment: BSQ_1

(b)   process variables
      t_{1-2}
      - intervention
      - duration of new hospitalization
      - security of attachment
      - parental support
        - sensitivity
        - parental attendance

(c)   posttest variables
      t_2
      - PHBQ
      - disturbed relationship
        - avoidance
        - negativity
      - BSQ_2

(d)   long-term follow-up
      t_3
      - BSQ_3
      - language
        - comprehension
        - expression
      - ego-resilience

The concept of *parental support* refers to *sensitivity and parental attendance* at the same time. Sensitivity and attendance are different, but related. A sizeable correlation of .59 was observed. It is one of our principal objectives to decide on the (relative) merits of parental attendance and sensitivity for prevention of upset and disturbance. To achieve this goal the two should be simultaneously entered as independent variables in ANCOVA. Another priority is the interaction of security and parental attendance as independent variables.

Parental attendance in the present report means the same as *parental presence or participation in hospital*. It is the pivotal variable of the study: one of the most important independent variables, but also the primary target of interventions and a criterion for their efficacy. Sensitivity *may be* an even more important dimension of parental support, but clearly has a different role on the stage. While promoting parental attendance might be a policy of some hospitals, promoting sensitivity would be a bridge too far.

(c)   *Posttest variables*

The general concept of posthospital adjustment refers to any measure of adjustment, either in the posttest or in the long-term follow-up. In the posttest three such measures are available:

PHBQ   is a criterion indicating changes labeled as upset, obtained by caregiver report one month after dicharge;

disturbed relationship   is a more specific measure of the adjustment between parent and child, obtained by observation, two months after discharge;

BSQ_2 is a general criterion of adjustment obtained from the caregiver, two months after discharge.

The measures supplement each other, because they represent different concepts and do not share the same sources of error. BSQ_2 is thought to be the best general measure of posthospital adjustment, but less sensitive to temporary influences. All three should be examined as dependent variables. The correlations among various measures of adjustment are found in Table 5.1. PHBQ and BSQ_2 correlated .50, but disturbance of relationship is correlated with neither. The two components of disturbed relationship: avoidance and negativity, intercorrelated .80.

TABLE 5.1   *Correlations among posthospital adjustment variables with pretest BSQ_1 included (N = 64)[1]*

		2	3	4	5	6
1.	BSQ_1	.17	.05	.59*	.40*	-.19
2.	PHBQ		-.02	.50*	.30*	-.02
3.	disturbed relationship			.13	.03	.07
4.	BSQ_2				.60*	-.30*
5.	BSQ_3					-.43*
6.	ego-resilience[1]					

[1]   for ego-resilience $n = 58$; for BSQ_3 $n = 62$; otherwise $n = 64$
[2]   * means $p<.05$

(d)   *long-term follow-up*

The late follow-up provides two general measures of adjustment: BSQ_3 and ego-resilience. They correlate -.43, as shown in Table 5.1. BSQ is a measure of disturbance and ego-resilience a measure of adaptedness. Both are relevant, but ego-resilience suffers from 6 missing values. Two measures of language development: comprehension and expression, are treated as a separate topic. Their correlation is .60.

Dichotomies

Most independent variables were split at the mean: BSQ_1 previous admissions, duration and sensitivity. For a skewed distribution like hospital days this means that the tail, including extremely high values, is selected as a category for comparison. This may be appropriate, as long as neither category is too small.

A specific choice was made for the variable parental attendance; the lower quartile was compared to the upper three quartiles. Impressions from the retrospective and prospective pilot studies suggested that differential effects on posthospital adjustment were to be found particularly for lower levels of parental attendance. Based on intuition, disturbance of relationship was dichotomized between the scores 3 and 4.

5.3   Influence of previous early hospitalization

A test on pretest adjustment

If early hospitalization is traumatic for many infants a part of the sample must be traumatized at t_1 , given their hospital records. This should manifest itself in BSQ_1, the measure of pretest adjustment. Cases with *more than one* previous admission are compared here to cases *without or with one* previous admission. Only previous admissions longer than one day are counted. Very early hospitalizations, because of deficiencies after birth or prematurity are included. Although at t_1 new surgery is scheduled this is not, for most children in the sample, a specific time of distress. Their previous hospitalization episode may be a few months or more than a year ago. The analysis with previous admissions as independent and age as covariate is displayed in Table 5.2.

For clinicians or researchers who believe long-term disturbance to be a common result, the outcome of ANCOVA shown in Table 5.2 is moderately reassuring. The adjustment of children without much of a hospitalization history is, at the time of pretest, somewhat better, but the difference in the two categories is not significant. Adjustment at time t_2 and t_3 is recorded here for the same categories of children. Additional testing, which is not relevant for the original hypothesis, shows that a small difference in BSQ_1 entails a significant difference in BSQ_2 and BSQ_3; it is a sign of vulnerability. Such differences should be discussed in connection with hypothesis (2).

A similar comparison was made with time spent in previous hospital episodes as independent variable. Twenty children had a hospitalization history longer than the mean of 22 days, with a maximum of 105 days. They were compared with 44 children below the mean. The results, displayed in Appendix 3.1, suggest that the time spent in hospital is *not* a predictor of (mal-)adjustment.

Hypothesis (1): *Prehospital adjustment will be related to hospitalization history: frequency and duration of preceding admissions,* is definitely not confirmed, although a "trend" was observed.

TABLE 5.2. *ANCOVA concerning effects of previous admissions on prehospital adjustment with age as covariate*

dependent variables[1]	previous admissions ≤ 1 $n = 39$		previous admissions > 1 $n = 25$			
	M	(SD)	M	(SD)	F	p^2
t_1 (pretest)						
BSQ$_1$	6.1	(4.4)	7.4	(4.3)	1.4	.12
t_2 (posttest)						
BSQ$_2$	5.6	(3.3)	7.9	(5.2)	4.6	.02
t_3 (long-term)						
BSQ$_3$[3]	6.3	(4.7)	8.4	(5.0)	3.0	.04

[1]   high score on BSQ indicate disadvantage
[2]   represents a one-sided probability
[3] $N = 62$ at t_3, otherwise $N = 64$

Previous hospitalization and vulnerability

It has been suggested that the experience of hospitalization may have a sensitizing effect. A sequence of readmissions may be much more disruptive than a single episode. The data in Table 5.2 seem to confirm this, because BSQ-scores after discharge, at time t_2 and t_3, are clearly elevated for history. Our second hypothesis proposes that this trend may be true for some infants/toddlers, but that opposite effects may apply for others. In the case of a new admission the psychological risk may be assessed by a combination of facts concerning adjustment at the time of admission and hospitalization history. Previous hospitalization may have had an effect similar to inoculation if adjustment at the time of readmission is satisfactory. If this hypothesis is true, vulnerability may be increased for some and decreased for others.

The hypothesis is tested by taking BSQ$_1$ (pretest) scores as criterion measure of adjustment at the time of admission. Those with BSQ$_1$ below the mean are designated insufficiently (re-)adjusted, and those with BSQ$_1$ above the mean as sufficiently (re-)adjusted. Both categories are next subdivided according to hospitalization history. Comparatively good adjustment is predicted specifically for children with good pretest adjustment, despite multiple hospitalizations. In Table 4.3 only interactional effects are tested. The *p*-values are adjusted for one-directional testing. If this ANCOVA, where BSQ$_1$ is entered as independent, is performed with BSQ$_2$ or BSQ$_3$ as criterion similar interactional effects are obvious, but these may be biased by any non-random common error variance of sequential BSQ-scores. Therefore only the PHBQ, disturbed relationship and ego-resilience were allowed as dependent variables. The result is shown in Table 5.3.

Table 5.3 provides support for hypothesis (2). Infants or toddlers with good pretest adjustment and multiple previous admissions have comparatively low PHBQ-scores and the lowest scores for disturbance of the relationship with their parent, while their scores for ego-resilience in the late follow-up are highest. Only for disturbed relationship the effect lacks significance. In fact the mean scores of these ten children are slightly better than the means of their counterparts with restricted hospitalization experience. So: *adequate adjustment, in spite of hospital experience indicates decreased or low vulnerability; prehospital maladjustment indicates increased vulnerability.* Hypothesis (2) is supported.

TABLE 5.3 *ANCOVA's with prehospital adjustment and previous admissions as factors and age as covariate. Dependent variables indicate posthospital adjustment.*

dependent variables[3]	BSQ$_1$ < 6.6 'sufficient (re-)adjustment'				BSQ$_1$ ≥ 6.6 'insufficient (re-)adjustment'					
	pre admi. ≤ 1 $n = 26$		pre admi. > 1 $n = 10$		pre admi. ≤ 1 $n = 13$		pre admi. > 1 $n = 15$			
	M	(SD)	M	(SD)	M	(SD)	M	(SD)	F[1]	p[2]
PHBQ	3.6	(4.6)	2.4	(3.1)	2.2	(3.8)	6.3	(5.5)	4.8	.02
disturbed relationship	3.2	(1.9)	2.6	(0.8)	3.4	(1.8)	4.0	(3.2)	1.1	.16
ego-resilience	.49	(.17)	.58	(.08)	.52	(.15)	.44	(.17)	4.0	.03

[1] *F* applies to interactional effects only. *df* (1,60)
[2] *p*-values represent a one-sided probability
[3] high scores on PHBQ and disturbed relationship indicate disadvantage; high scores on ego-resilience indicate advantage
[4] *N* = 58 for ego-resilience

5.4   Effect of interventions

Effect of interventions on parental support

In Section 3.3 interventions were distinguished as 'true interventions' ($n = 25$) or 'tentative interventions'. Four interventions were classified as tentative because the consultant felt that her approach had to be improved by experience at the time. It was agreed that a test of efficacy should exclude tentative interventions. The effect of interventions on parental attendance is tested by ANCOVA, while number of previous admissions and age were entered as possibly relevant covariates. The ANCOVA results are displayed in Table 5.4.

Table 5.4 shows that interventions have significantly stimulated parental attendance. Further analysis has indicated that each of the nine items in the scale of parental attendance has contributed to this effect, with *nights of rooming-in (proportional)* on top of the bill. The total effect size is 2.9 scale points, which amounts to an effect size of .47, about half a standard

deviation of the total distribution. Hypothesis (3): *Interventions directed towards parents will enhance parental support, manifest as*
- *longer presence at daytime in hospital*
- *more frequent rooming-in at night*
- *more frequent presence at induction of anaesthesia*
- *more involvement of father,*

is thus supported, with the reservation that *specific* effects mentioned here can not be affirmed with the same confidence as the general (pooled) effect.

TABLE 5.4   *ANCOVA for effect of interventions on parental presence, with age and previous admissions as covariates*

dependent variable	no intervention $n = 35$		true intervention $n = 25$			
	M	(SD)	M	(SD)	F^2	p^1
parental presence	-1.3	(6.7)	1.6	(4.9)	4.1	.02
standard error of mean			1.1		1.0	

1	*p* represents a one-sided probability
2	*df* (1 , 56)

Effect of interventions on upset and disturbance

While interventions were aimed at enhancement of parental support, the ultimate goal was, of course, to prevent upset and/or disturbance of the child. The attainment of this goal is dependent upon the magnitude of differences in parental support caused by interventions, as well as on the effect of such a difference upon adjustment of the child. The existence of this indirect effect, proposed in hypothesis (4) is tested here by ANCOVA on general measures of adjustment at short- and long-term follow-up. The results are displayed in Table 5.5.

The outcome is clearly negative. Hypothesis (4): *posthospital upset and maladjustment will be reduced by interventions,* is not supported by the data.

TABLE 5.5   *ANCOVAs for effect of interventions on subsequent posthospital adjustment of the child. Previous admissions, age and prehospital adjustment (BSQ₁) are employed as covariates*

time of measurement[1]	dependent variables[2]	no intervention $n = 35$		true intervention $n = 25$			
		M	(SD)	M	(SD)	F[3]	p[4]
t_1	BSQ_1	5.9	(3.9)	6.8	(4.4)	(pretest)	
t_{1-2}	PHBQ	2.9	(4.2)	5.0	(5.2)	2.9	.09
t_2	BSQ_2	5.9	(3.7)	7.0	(4.9)	.2	.63
t_2	disturbed relationship	3.4	(2.5)	3.2	(1.8)	.4	.76
t_3	BSQ_3	6.5	(4.7)	8.1	(5.2)	.2	.66
t_3	ego-resilience[5]	.52	(.16)	.46	(.16)	1.8	.18

[1] t_1 = time of pretest; t_{1-2} = one month after discharge; t_2 = 2 months after discharge, t_3 = late follow-up
[2] high scores on ego-resilience indicate advantage; otherwise high scores indicate disadvantage
[3] df (1 , 55)
[4] p-values represent two-sided probabilities
[5] n = 58 for ego-resilience; df (1 , 53)

5.5   Further antecedent conditions of upset and disturbance

Effects of duration of admissions

First a test is performed for the effect of the time spent in hospital on subsequent adjustment. The number of hospital days required for the selected admissions ranges from 5 to 25, including the day of discharge. The mean is 11.0. Posthospital adjustment means for short and long admissions are reported in Table 5.6, where the prehospital BSQ_1, although not a dependent variable, is included. The F-test indicates no significant differences. So hypothesis (5): *posthospital adjustment will be related to duration of a new admission,* is not confirmed by any outcome measure.

TABLE 5.6 *ANCOVA for effect of duration of hospitalization on subsequent adjustment, with previous admissions, age and prehospital adjustment (BSQ_1) as covariates*

| | | duration 5-10 days | | duration 11-25 days | | | |
| | | n = 36 | | n = 28 | | | |
dependent variables[1]		M	(SD)	M	(SD)	F^2	p^3
$t_1{}^4$	BSQ_1	7.3	(4.0)	5.7	(4.7)	(pretest)	
t_{1-2}	PHBQ	4.1	(4.2)	3.3	(5.2)	.4	.51
t_2	BSQ_2	6.8	(4.0)	6.1	(4.3)	.5	.50
t_2	disturbed relationship	3.3	(2.3)	3.4	(2.1)	.1	.79
t_3	BSQ_3	7.6	(5.)	6.5	(4.7)	.8	.94
t_3	ego resilience[5]	.51	(.13)	.47	(.18)	1.2	.27

[1] high scores indicate a disadvantage, except for ego-resilience
[2] $df (1 , 57)$
[3] p-values represent two-sided probabilities
[4] time of measurement is explained sub Table 5.5
[5] $n = 58$ for ego-resilience

Effects of parental support

To consider possible effects of parental support, the descriptive statistics of adjustment scores are compared for the dichotomies of attendance and sensitivity in Table 5.7. For BSQ_1 the means are exactly as might be predicted: no difference for parental attendance, because the hospitalization has not yet occurred; some difference for sensitivity which represents a stable feature of the home environment. For PHBQ the means are contrary to expectation and prediction: it seems as if parental attendance in hospital augments short-term upset, while effects of sensitivity on maladjustment are nearly zero. No effect is recorded for BSQ_2: posttest means are nearly identical to pretest means. Conspicuously different are the findings for disturbance of relationship (two months after discharge), which are in the predicted direction for both support variables. Even more surprising (after the absence of any effect on BSQ_2) is the difference among cell means of BSQ_3, for both support variables. This difference in posthospital adjustment has arisen among the 16 subjects where parental attendance was comparatively low. Their disturbance scores have become elevated at t_3, while the majority, with proper parental attendance, is still at the pretest level. The same sort of effect is suggested by the means of ego-resilience, both for parental attendance and sensitivity. The observed differences are fairly small, however.

Before proceeding with hypothesis testing it should be noted that throughout the analysis similar patterns were observed for the relationship between a set of process variables that represents a specific hypothesis and the collection of criterion measures. The pattern is that changes as predicted may be observed at t_3, mainly as a predicted long-term effect on BSQ_3, but weakly reflected by ego-resilience scores. At t_2 a similar effect may be found for disturbance of relationship, but not for BSQ_2, while for PHBQ some opposite effects are found. In the course of our exposition we will try to describe, understand and explain such results.

The test for a beneficial effect of parental support should be done first with both parental attendance and sensitivity as simultaneous independent variables. ANCOVAs have been performed. This produced a significant result for disturbed relationship, but insignificant *F*-

TABLE 5.7   *Descriptive statistics concerning possible effects of parental presence in hospital and sensitivity of parents on subsequent adjustment of the child*

		parental presence				sensitivity[1]			
		'low'		'medium/high'		below mean		above mean	
		n = 16		n = 48		n = 26		n = 27	
dependent variable[2]		M	(SD)	M	(SD)	M	(SD)	M	(SD)
t_1[3]	BSQ$_1$	6.8	(4.7)	6.5	(4.3)	7.1	(4.8)	5.4	(4.1)
t_{1-2}	PHBQ	2.6	(3.8)	4.1	(4.7)	3.2	(5.0)	3.8	(4.5)
t_2	BSQ$_2$	6.8	(3.4)	6.4	(4.5)	6.8	(4.8)	5.7	(4.1)
t_2	dis.relationship	4.7	(3.2)	2.9	(1.5)	4.2	(2.9)	2.7	(1.3)
t_3	BSQ$_3$	8.8	(5.9)	6.5	(4.4)	7.8	(4.8)	6.5	(5.6)
t_3	ego-resilience	.46	(.15)	.51	(.16)	.46	(.16)	.50	(.16)

[1]   eleven cases with missing values for sensitivity are left out of this comparison
[2]   high scores indicate disadvantage, except for ego-resilience
[3]   time of measurement is explained sub Table 5.5

values for all other dependent variables. To simplify the multitude of tables, the tables 5.8, 5.10 and 5.12 are limited to disturbed relationship and BSQ$_3$ as dependent variables. Table 5.8 represents effects of parental support.

Just one effect is significant: the main effect of parental presence on disturbance of the relationship. This shows an increase of disturbance in the relationship for lower levels of parental presence. No interactional effects are observed; sensitivity and presence may contribute independently to the adjustment of the toddler. If sensitivity prevents disturbances in the relationship, then this contribution is not large enough to appear significant in our sample (which may be due to eleven cases with missing values). Hypothesis (6): *Posthospital adjustment will be related to parental support: parental presence and sensitivity,* has acquired very limited support, suggesting that parental presence in hospital goes some way to prevent disturbance of relationship.

TABLE 5.8   *ANCOVA-results for effect of parental presence and sensitivity on disturbed relationship and BSQ$_3$ with previous admissions, age and prehospital adjustment as covariates*

| | disturbed relationship[1] | | | BSQ$_3$[1] | | |
	F	(df)	p	F	(df)	p
main effect:						
parental presence	5.3	(1,55)	.04	2.2	(1,53)	.15
main effect:						
sensitivity[2]	2.3	(2,55)	.11	.1	(2,53)	.90
interaction:						
parental presence						
x sensitivity	.6	(2,55)	.55	1.3	(2,53)	.28

[1]   for disturbed relationship n = 64; for BSQ$_3$ n = 62
[2]   eleven cases with missing values for sensitivity were entered as a separate category in the analysis

84

Effects of attachment-quality after hospitalization

In Table 5.9 means and standard deviations of dependent variables among (initially) securely attached and (initially) insecurely attached infants can be compared.

TABLE 5.9   *Descriptive statistics for prehospital adjustment and posthospital adjustment related to security of attachment*

	adjustment variables	insecure $n = 22$		secure $n = 37$	
		M	(SD)	M	(SD)
t_1	BSQ_1	8.0	(5.6)	6.1	(3.6)
t_{1-2}	PHBQ	3.4	(4.4)	3.9	(4.7)
t_2	BSQ_2	6.3	(4.8)	6.7	(4.1)
t_2	dis. relationship	3.4	(1.7)	3.3	(2.3)
t_3	BSQ_3	6.0	(4.5)	7.8	(5.2)
t_3	ego-resilience	.48	(.14)	.50	(.18)

The differences are not very large and definitely fail to support the hypothesis (7): *Quality of attachment will modify posthospital adjustment; maladjustment will be more likely when attachment is insecure.* The remarkable feature of Table 5.9 is that, while securely attached infants are better adjusted at t_1, judging by their lower BSQ_1 scores, they have slightly higher BSQ_2 scores and distinctly higher BSQ_3 scores.

The effect of security should be evaluated in connection with the effect of attendance. The ANCOVAs for this topic with disturbed relationship and BSQ_3 as dependent variables are reported in Table 5.10. The results are remarkable: sizeable F-values that should be interpreted with caution because they represent unpredicted effects. At least, the direction of the main effect of security and the interactions with parental presence are unpredicted (and therefore not significant). The dynamics of the process are more clearly revealed in Table 5.11. Apparently eight infants who were initially[1] securely attached, but who experienced limited (insufficient) parental presence (first row of the table) have high scores for disturbance of the relationship with their parent and very high scores for BSQ_3. In contrast, 29 securely attached children that received sufficient parental attendance, have low scores for disturbance on both criteria. Insecurely attached infants seem to adapt better to a comparatively low degree of parental support.

The main effect of parental attendance provides support for hypothesis (6); this effect is of true significance, even for BSQ_3. Hypothesis (7): *Quality of attachment will modify posthospital adjustment; upset will be more likely when attachment is insecure,* is supported as regards the first part but refuted as regards the second part of the statement. Securely attached infants are vulnerable. The results suggest that parental presence in the hospital is of vital importance for them. Of course the conclusion that secure attachment cannot be conceived of as a protective factor, is dependent on the validity of classification, discussed in Sections 4.4 and 7.1.

---

[1]   A follow-up measure for quality of attachment is not available; disturbed relationship does not necessarily mean insecure attachment.

TABLE 5.10   *ANCOVA-results for effect of parental presence and security on disturbed relationship and BSQ$_3$ with previous admissions, age and prehospital adjustment as covariates*

	disturbed relationship[1]			BSQ$_3$[1]		
	F	(df)	p	F	(df)	p
main effect:						
parental presence	7.2	(1,55)	.01	3.3	(1.53)	.08
main effect:						
security[2]	.5	(2,55)	.60	4.8	(2,53)	.01[3]
interaction:						
parental presence x security	4.1	(2,55)	.02[3]	2.4	(2,53)	.10

[1]   for disturbed relationship $n = 64$; for BSQ$_3$ $n = 62$
[2]   five cases with missing values for security were entered as a separate category in the analysis
[3]   although $p < .05$ this effect is not significant, because the direction of the effect runs counter to prediction

TABLE 5.11   *Descriptive statistics for possible influences of attachment quality and parental attendance upon posthospital adjustment and interactional effects*

factor levels of quality of attachment and parental presence		dependent variables				adjusted[2]	
		disturbed relationship		BSQ$_3$		BSQ$_3$	
	n	M	(SD)	M	(SD)	M	(SD)
secure							
parental presence 'low'	8	4.9	(4.0)	12.6	(4.0)	8.1	(4.6)
parental presence 'medium/high'	29	2.8	(1.3)	6.4[1]	(4.7)	2.4[1]	(3.1)
insecure							
parental presence 'low'	7	3.7	(1.3)	5.0	(5.4)	1.1	(3.8)
parental presence 'medium/high'	15	3.2	(2.0)	6.4	(4.1)	2.6	(3.7)
entire sample	64	3.3	(2.2)	7.1	(4.9)	3.2	(3.9)

[1] $n = 27$
[2]   the adjusted BSQ$_3$ is the residual when BSQ$_2$ has been partialled out; high values indicate deterioration

Interactional effects of duration and parental presence

It was hypothesized that the difference between low parental attendance and high parental attendance might be magnified if a child was kept in hospital longer. No influence of duration was found in Table 5.6 but some effect might be found in interactional effects. This was tested in two ANCOVA's, where parental presence and duration simultaneously served as independent variables, while disturbed relationship and BSQ_3 were consecutive dependents. The outcomes are presented in Table 5.12.

TABLE 5.12   ANCOVAs for interactional effects of duration and parental presence on posthospital adjustment, with age, previous admissions and BSQ_1 as covariates

	disturbed relationship			BSQ_3		
	F	(df)	p	F	(df)	p
main effect						
parental presence	6.1	(1,55)	.02	2.6	(1,55)	.11
main effect						
duration	.0	(1,55)	.87	.1	(1,55)	.79
interaction						
presence x duration	2.5	(1,55)	.12	.3	(1,55)	.61

In Table 5.12 no significant interactional effects are found. A significant main effect confirms the general relevance of parental presence. The hypothesis (8): *duration of admission and parental presence will exhibit interactional effects*, is not supported.

Avoidance and negativity

As explained in Section 3.3 the construct *disturbed relationship* was defined as the sum of *avoidant behavior* and *negativity* on the part of the child, while playing with the mother in the posttest session, two months after discharge. Within the context of attachment theory it is important to know the expression of any disturbance of the relationship. In Section 1.3 reasons were given to expect *avoidant behavior* after hospitalization with less than satisfactory parental attendance, a conjecture formulated as hypothesis (9).

A separate ANCOVA was performed with the two components of disturbed relationship as consecutive dependent variables; the independent one was parental attendance in both cases.

Table 5.13 demonstrates that both dependent variables are affected by parental attendance. Thus hypothesis (9): *Lack of parental attendance will disturb the child-caregiver*

TABLE 5.13   ANCOVA's for main effects of parental presence on the separate components of disturbed relationship: avoidance and negativity, with age, previous admissions and BSQ_1 as covariates

	parental presence 'low' $n = 16$		parental presence 'medium/high' $n = 48$			
dependent variable	M	(SD)	M	(SD)	$F(1,60)$	p
avoidance	2.6	(1.6)	1.6	(1.0)	6.1	.02
negativity	2.1	(1.7)	1.3	(.6)	6.3	.02

relationship, specifically increase avoidant behavior, is confirmed. The addition "specifically" should perhaps be left out, because negativity may be expected as well.

The relationship of upset and long-term disturbance

It was hypothesized that long-term disturbance should be related to the same predictors as short-term upset. This is definitely not the case. BSQ_3 was taken as the primary criterion of long-term disturbance, PHBQ as the primary criterion of short-term upset. Although the two measures correlate .30 they are not influenced or predicted in the same way by the aspects of hospitalization or parent-child-interaction studied here. On the contrary: it was found that upset *as measured by the PHBQ* tended to be increased by parental support, while BSQ_3 tended to decrease; a finding which will be critically evaluated in Section 7.1.

BSQ_2 which might be considered as a measure of posthospital upset different from PHBQ was strongly related to BSQ_3 by a correlation of .60, but did not reflect effects of the same predictors, like parental support. Disturbed relationship may be a symptom of posthospital upset, but it is a much more specific construct. Hypothesis (10) is therefore devoid of any support, but in Section 7.1 this state of affairs is interpreted as an artifact.

5.6   Hospitalization and language development

With the help of the manual (Reynell & Huntley, 1977) the scores were expressed as age levels: the age in months when the observed performance may be expected according to the norms. These scores were divided by chronological age. The norms applied here are British and not up to date. Therefore the scores are considered valid for comparisons within the sample, but not for any comparison to external standards. The mean of obtained comprehension quotients was 95 ($SD = 21$), the mean and *SD* of expression quotients the same. Children within the upper quartile of the BSQ_3 distribution have a mean comprehension quotient of 86 ($SD = 19$) and a mean expression quotient of 87 ($SD = 18$), which suggests that their language development has been impaired by general adjustment problems. Table 5.14 serves to present in a systematic way some differences of language development in relation to previous conditions.

Language development will be dependent on many conditions other than those considered here. The relationship between various independent variables and language development was not expected to be strong. However, parental support is expected to influence this behavioral domain as well as general adjustment. This is borne out by Table 5.14.

According to the data presented here, sensitivity at time t_{1-2} is the best predictor of achievements in comprehension and expression at t_3, while disturbed (t_2) relationship also seems to be relevant in predicting delay or underachievement. Again the significance of such influences is investigated here by testing pairs of independents. In Table 5.15 the two support-measures: sensitivity and attendance during hospitalization are entered simultaneously. The impact of sensitivity is strongly confirmed, while the effect of presence in hospital is "absorbed" by it. In a few cases with satisfactory sensitivity and comparatively low presence the language development is unperturbed.

This outcome makes sense, seeing sensitivity as a continuous influence and presence in hospital an episode.

TABLE 5.14 *Descriptive statistics concerning possible influences of early conditions on language development*

	n	comprehension quotient		expression quotient	
		M	(SD)	M	(SD)
previous admissions					
≤ 1	39	95	(22)	97	(19)
2 - 6	25	94	(20)	91	(24)
attachment quality					
secure	35	94	(19)	91	(21)
insecure	22	96	(25)	99	(23)
sensitivity					
below mean	25	85	(13)	84	(14)
above mean	26	104	(18)	98	(25)
parental presence					
low	16	91	(25)	92	(19)
medium/high	46	96	(20)	95	(22)
disturbed relationship					
≤ 3	43	99	(22)	97	(22)
> 3	19	85	(13)	90	(20)

TABLE 5.15 *ANCOVAs for effect of sensitivity and presence in hospital on language development with age, previous admissions and prehospital adjustment as covariates*

		n	comprehension quotient		expression quotient	
			M	(SD)	M	(SD)
sensitivity below mean						
parental presence 'low'		10	81	(14)	83	(16)
parental presence 'medium/high'		15	87	(12)	85	(13)
sensitivity above mean						
parental presence 'low'		3	117	(8)	115	(4)
parental presence 'medium/high'		23	103	(18)	101	(23)
main effect sensitivity			$F_{(2,53)} = 6.3$		$F_{(2,53)} = 4.7$	
	p-value		.00		.01	
main effect parental presence			$F_{(2,53)} = .3$		$F_{(2,53)} = .1$	
	p-value		.61		.74	
sensitivity x parental presence			$F_{(2,53)} = 1.7$		$F_{(2,53)} = .5$	
	p-value		.18		.61	

To limit the number of tables in the present chapter, ANCOVAs with other pairs of independent variables will be included as appendices:
- number of previous admissions x parental presence: Appendix 3.2
- attachment quality x parental presence: Appendix 3.3
- attachment quality x disturbed relationship: Appendix 3.4

The results contained in those tables will be, of course, presented here. Although hospitalization history in itself is not a predictor of language development, a significant interactional effect is found with parental presence: six cases with multiple episodes in hospital and low parental attendance are seriously delayed, both in comprehension and expression (Appendix 3.2).

Attachment quality and parental presence, the pair of predictors that was earlier found to modify general adjustment, did not yield significant effects on language development. Both main effects and interactional effects proved to be insignificant (Appendix 3.3). This negative result raised the question whether disturbance of relationship might be irrelevant to language development. This question was answered by entering attachment quality and disturbed relationship in one ANCOVA (Appendix 3.4). A strong main effect of disturbed relationship on development of language comprehension was established; impact on expressive language and interactional effects were not significant.

The original hypothesis (11): *Speech or language acquisition will be related to the same predictors as posthospital adjustment* can not be maintained in its original form. Although speech development is found to be dependent on parental support, it is the sensitivity dimension of support that counts most, not the conditions of hospitalization. At the same time, a combination of repeated hospitalization and poor parental attendance can, according to our findings, disrupt language development. The general conclusion is that hospitalization history will impair language acquisition if adverse conditions prevail. In such conditions general adjustment and language development may be simultaneously affected.

5.7   Summing up

A number of unexpected results were obtained, while a number of hypotheses was disconfirmed. It was found that no effects of parental support either from presence in the hospital or from sensitivity could be found in the PHBQ-scores or BSQ_2-scores. For PHBQ-scores effects were contrary to expectations: the data suggested negative effects of parental support in hospital. Clearly hypothesis (10), that predicted similar effects for short-term follow-up and long-term follow-up had to be abandoned. This negative finding complicates final judgement concerning hypotheses that were confirmed.

The main effect of hospitalization history on preadmission adjustment was not significant, therefore hypothesis (1) was not confirmed. In this case, however, the effect was in the direction predicted, suggesting that preadmission adjustment (BSQ_1) might be affected by hospitalization history, but not strongly.

Hypothesis (2), suggesting that vulnerability might be gauged by a combination of data on previous hospitalizations and preadmission adjustment, was firmly supported.

An effect of interventions on parental presence, predicted by hypothesis (3), was confirmed. The effects on posthospital adjustment of the child, predicted by hypothesis (4) were not found.

Hypothesis (5) presumed that posthospital adjustment would be related to duration of the hospital episode; it was disconfirmed. Posthospital adjustment was related to parental support as predicted by hypothesis (6). Of the two aspects of parental support: sensitivity and presence in hospital, only the latter was found to be a significant predictor of general adjustment at the time of late follow-up.

In Hypothesis (7) quality of attachment was conjectured to be a protective factor. The results indicated that this was not the case: subsequent adjustment of initially securely attached infants was average in the case of sufficient parental presence, but damaged if parental presence was comparatively low.

A significant interaction of duration and parental presence, as specified in hypothesis (8) was not confirmed. Parental presence did influence disturbance of the relationship, however: insufficient parental presence enhanced avoidant behavior, as suggested in hypothesis (9).

Hypothesis (11), concerning effects of the hospital episode on language development, was partially confirmed. Scores of disturbed relationship were related to language acquisition, but sensitivity was the best predictor of language development, both of comprehension and of expression.

CHAPTER 6 DESCRIPTION OF DATA REGARDING ROOMING-IN, DIAGNOSIS AND DEGREE OF DISTURBANCE BY HOSPITALIZATION

In the present chapter, various findings not involved in hypothesis testing are presented. In Section 6.1 a specific form of parental support, rooming-in, will be considered. In Section 6.2 dependent variables will be related to the diagnosis that was the ultimate reason for surgery. In Section 6.3 the degree of developmental damage in the poulation that can reasonably attributed to hospitalization is estimated. Developmental disturbance will be the central concept and specific BSQ-problems of children in the sample will be distinguished.

6.1   Effects of rooming-in

In previous chapters the subject of parental presence in hospital was treated with some special emphasis on rooming-in. As far as one can judge by previously accumulated knowledge, rooming-in should be strongly recommended. An impression of the possible effects of rooming-in from data collected in the present study is afforded by the data of Table 6.1.

TABLE 6.1   *Posthospital adjustment related to rooming-in*

time of measurement	dependent variable	no rooming-in $n = 23$		partial rooming-in $n = 21$		full rooming-in $n = 20$	
		M	(SD)	M	(SD)	M	(SD)
t_1	BSQ_1	5.7	(4.6)	6.6	(5.0)	7.6	(3.4)
t_2	disturbed rel.	4.1	(3.0)	3.3	(1.9)	2.6	(0.9)
t_2	BSQ_2	4.9	(3.4)	6.5	(4.4)	8.3	(4.5)
t_3	BSQ_3	7.0	(5.5)	6.3	(4.7)	8.1	(4.3)

In Tables 6.1 and 6.2 a selection of dependent variables is considered, because in the preceding analyses two variables emerged as most sensitive to possible causes of disturbance: disturbed relationship and BSQ_3. BSQ_3-scores are naturally interpreted most accurately in relation to BSQ_2 and BSQ_1-scores. The variable disturbed relationship is sandwiched in the tables between BSQ-measurements to preserve the chronological order.

Table 6.1 provides partial support for the protective value of rooming-in. BSQ_3-scores are highest for children with full rooming-in, but the same difference is found for BSQ_1-scores. Apparently poor preadmission adjustment of a child is one factor which may make parents choose rooming-in. An effect of rooming-in on long-term adjustment is not apparent from Table 6.1. Disturbance of the relationship at t_2 , however, is less if rooming-in is practiced. The opinion that partial rooming-in may be a very poor choice (voiced by one parent who happened to be a professional nurse) is not reinforced by the present data.

The potential of rooming-in to prevent disturbance of relationship was conjectured to be stronger within the group of patients admitted for the first time than within the sample as a whole. This hunch has been confirmed by computing the point biserial correlation between rooming-in (scored 1 for any night or 0 for not at all) and disturbance of relationship. This correlation turned out to be -.26 ($p < .05$) in the whole sample and -.45 ($p < .05$) for patients without prior hospital experience.

6.2   Possible implications of diagnosis for long-term adjustment

The possibility that some diseases may have consequences for long-term psychological adjustment can be admitted without empirical proof. This may be true for some conditions that entail, for instance, frequent readmissions, a program of surgical interventions and/or severe restrictions on normal behavior like long-term plaster-casts. Not much is known, however, about the relationship of particular problems to later development. The present data yield some factual information, which should be reported in spite of serious limitations. An objection to statistical comparisons between diagnostic categories is the confounding in our data of diagnosis and the setting of the treatment. Obviously experts on specific types of surgery are not equally divided among hospitals. In many cases a specific hospital had been selected because of the specialized surgeon, irrespective of the distance.

Three diagnostic categories were selected for comparison because of sufficient size:

17 cases of *hypospadia*: patients from hospital I and III, a fairly homogeneous category with a comparatively short hospitalization history;

17 cases of serious *gastro-intestinal* problems requiring surgery, recruited in 4 different hospitals: I, II, III and V. This category includes 3 cases of Hirschsprung's disease with extended hospitalization histories, 3 cases of anus atresia, and various other problems;

10 cases of *heart diseases*, patients of hospital III and IV: 4 cases with Tetralogy of Fallot, 6 cases with atrium septum defects of the second type (ASD II).

The hospitals are referred to by arbitrary numerals because it is not their identity which is important here, but the degree of confounding. In spite of our caveat, Table 6.2, which suggests differences of adjustment of these categories, may be of interest. In this table the total

TABLE 6.2   *Posthospital adjustment related to disease category*

variables:	(1) hypo-spadia $n = 17$		(2) gastro-intestinal $n = 17$		(3) cong. heart disease $n = 10$		entire sample $N = 64$	
	M	(SD)	M	(SD)	M	(SD)	M	(SD)
total time in hospital	22	(22)	48	(32)	30	(27)	34	(30)
t_1 BSQ$_1$	6.2	(4.5)	6.7	(4.6)	7.2	(4.0)	6.6	(4.4)
t_2 disturbed relationship	2.9	(1.2)	3.6	(2.6)	2.6	(1.1)	3.3	(2.2)
t_2 BSQ$_2$	5.5	(3.7)	6.8	(4.8)	5.8	(3.5)	6.5	(4.3)
t_3 BSQ$_3$	5.6	(5.7)	7.8	(5.3)	10.0	(4.9)	7.1	(4.9)

number of days spent in hospital is recorded as a descriptive feature. The total number of days includes any admission form birth till the late follow-up.There are substantial differences in long-term adjustment between the diagnostic categories in Table 6.2. The impact of genital surgery is found to be a minor threat to general (behavioral) adjustment. As expected, the final outcome for gastro-intestinal cases is worse, which may be explained by their long and cumbersome medical histories, visible in a mean of 48 hospital days. Many of these children, and their parents, have been burdened by recurrent severe complaints and practical assignments like hygienic care with an Anus Praeter (an artificial route for defaecation) for considerable periods.

The early scores of patients with heart diseases seem to be moderate, but the mean score of 10 points for BSQ_3 is exceptionally high. The most salient item among various behavioral problems is an increase in fits of anger in the course of the first year after surgery.

Because of their small number, four cases with congenital luxation of hips were not included in Table 6.2. This category was conspicuous at the time of data collection because of hospitalization history, the suffering imposed by immobilization and the problems reported by parents. The mean BSQ_3 of these children was equal to that of patients with heart diseases.

6.3   Long-term disturbance indicated by the BSQ

The question at the heart of our inquiry is the degree of developmental disturbance that can be attributed to hospitalization experiences. This cannot be judged from a single statistic, even when one instrument, the BSQ, is chosen for a criterion. Because of its stability and validity the BSQ is considered the best available criterion for long-term development. The increase in BSQ-scores from pretest to t_3 is a first approximation. To quantify the difference an effect size formula devised by Cohen (1977) can be utilized:

$$d_{31} = \frac{M_3 - M_1}{\sigma_1 \sqrt{1 - r_{13}}}$$

For this case we estimate σ, the population standard deviation in Cohen's formula, by the pretest standard deviation. Thus the effect is

$$d_{31} = \frac{7.1 - 6.6}{4.4 \sqrt{1 - .40}}$$

$$d_{31} = .15$$

Seeing .20 is designated as 'small' in Cohen's conventional definition, .15 can hardly be called a severe degree of deterioration. At the same time we know that emotional and behavioral problems can be very serious and upsetting in *individual* instances. Both perspectives: that of the individual case and of the population are relevant.

It may be questioned whether the effect size just calculated represents effects of hospitalization. In fact it is the result of everything which happened between t_1 and t_3, including maturation. Therefore the effect, uncorrected by any comparison with nonhospitalized subjects, is not a pure hospitalization effect (it might turn out to be larger or smaller). On the other hand, statistical analyses in Chapter 5 have demonstrated that BSQ_3 scores could be predicted from conditions of hospitalization, like parental presence, at least to some extent.

A second approximation of this degree of disturbance is found by concentrating on subsamples with different levels of parental presence. A remarkable feature of those with a medium or high level of parental presence is that the means of their BSQ_1-scores and BSQ_3-scores are exactly equal: 6.5 (compare Table 5.7). At the same time the mean scores of those with comparatively low parental presence have risen from 6.8 at t_1 to 8.8 at t_3. The effect size can be calculated as

$$ d_{31} = \frac{8.8 - 6.8}{4.7 \sqrt{1 - .40}} = 0.59 $$

Seeing .50 designated a 'medium' effect-size in Cohen's conventional definition, .59 is a sizeable effect. This figure has some meaning in relation to the effect size of .15 for the entire sample and .00 for those with satisfactory parental attendance: the deterioration in this group is presumably caused by the conditions of hospitalization, certainly not by maturation, probably not by accidental circumstance.

Another way to describe the same effect is an observation made while studying a listing of the sample. Among the sixty-four cases, six can be found with the following pattern:
- the score for maladjustment at t_3 (BSQ_3) is high: 1.4 to 2.0 standard deviations above the mean
- the score for maladjustment represents an increase: it is at least (at the time of the late follow-up) twice as large as the pretest score
- the score for parental presence is low, it is at least one standard deviation below the mean

Such cases can be counted as victims of long-term developmental disturbance due to hospitalization with insufficient parental support, without denying the complexity of developmental and interactional processes involved here.

The change in BSQ-scores is the sum of changes concerning particular areas of behavior, earlier called topics. Of course we are interested to know which topics are involved, either by an increase or by a decrease in the time span between t_1 and t_3. When investigating these topics it should be borne in mind that changes in behavior are not the ultimate target of inquiry and prevention. Behavioral changes may be a problem in themselves, they represent another problem: emotional distress and long-term damage of confidence. This maladaptive change is the proper target of prevention. The changes in mean scores for particular topics are summarized in Table 6.3.

From Table 6.3 four topics can be identified as showing an increase: (1) noncompliance; (2) attention seeking; (3) moodiness; (4) sleeping with parents. The second topic, attention seeking, is identical to the most frequently found posthospitalization characteristic in our retrospective research, where a nonhospitalized sample was used for comparison. 'Sleeping with parents' (sometimes, not necessarily whole nights or every night) is similarly to be regarded as a specific symptom. In other topics some maturation effect may be involved. (An estimate of maturation effects can be obtained by correlation of BSQ-items with age. A table of relevant correlations is included as Appendix 3.5. It is found that age correlates positively with noncompliance and attention seeking at t_1 and t_2; at t_3 the correlations have reverted to zero. Correlations of age with total BSQ are negligible, at any time.) A substantial increase in

TABLE 6.3   *Increase and decrease of specific behavior problems between pretest and late follow-up in whole sample (N = 62)*

Problem Behavior[1]	t_1 M_1	(SD)	t_3 M_3	(SD)	Cohen's d d	
bedtime resistance	.44	(.75)	.60	(.90)	.28	
waking in the night	.78	(.93)	.69	(.93)	-.12	
sleeping with parents	.28	(.58)	.48	(.84)	.45	!
overactivity	.56	(.69)	.56	(.69)	.00	
poor concentration	.55	(.66)	.48	(.67)	-.14	
trouble with peers	.17	(.49)	.24	(.56)	.18	
attention seeking	.73	(.80)	1.08	(.75)	.56	!
separation protest	.61	(.79)	.34	(.72)	-.44	
rejection of babysitter	.30	(.55)	.05	(.22)	-.59	
noncompliance	.34	(.57)	.63	(.71)	.66	!
fits of anger	.45	(.56)	.58	(.67)	.30	
moody	.05	(.28)	.16	(.45)	.51	!
fearful	.59	(.66)	.56	(.74)	-.06	
eating problem	.73	(.78)	.65	(.63)	-.13	
Total BSQ	6.59	(4.39)	7.11	(4.88)	.15	
habits	1.50	(1.51)	1.10	(1.29)	-.34	

[1]   ! indicates effect sizes > .40

noncompliance is found, but it should not entirely be attributed to hospitalization. To complete the exploration of behavior difficulties a similar table is presented for those with lower parental attendance: Table 6.4.

In Table 6.4 five topics are identified that show a substantial increase. The largest effect size is found for noncompliance, other items are: sleeping with parents, bedtime resistance, attention seeking and overactivity. Large effects in comparison to what was found in the sample as a whole can not logically be attributed to maturation.

The symptoms reported here do not give a true insight into developmental disturbances manifested in individual cases with severe problems. For that purpose a more elaborate individual case description is indispensable.

TABLE 6.4   *Increase and decrease in specific behavior problems between pretest and late follow-up in subsample with lower parental attendance (n = 16)*

Problem Behavior[1]	t_1 M_1	(SD)	t_3 M_3	(SD)	d	
bedtime resistance	.44	(.81)	1.13	(.96)	1.10	!
waking in the night	.88	(.89)	.63	(.89)	-.36	
sleeping with parents	.19	(.54)	.75	(1.00)	1.34	!
overactivity	.63	(.72)	.31	(.60)	.57	!
poor concentration	.50	(.73)	.56	(.81)	.11	
trouble with peers	.37	(.72)	.31	(.70)	-.11	
attention seeking	.75	(.68)	1.13	(.72)	.72	!
separation protest	.50	(.82)	.56	(.89)	.09	
rejection of babysitter	.44	(.63)	.13	(.34)	-.64	
noncompliance	.19	(.40)	1.06	(.68)	2.81	!
fits of anger	.50	(.52)	.63	(.72)	.32	
moody	.00	(.00)	.19	(.40)	--	
fearful	.69	(.79)	.56	(.73)	-.21	
eating problem	.75	(.77)	.81	(.50)	.10	
Total BSQ	6.81	(4.65)	8.75	(5.93)	.54	!
habits	1.69	(1.30)	1.38	(1.26)	-.31	

[1]   ! indicates effect sizes > .40

6.4   Summing up

From the analyses it may be concluded that rooming-in serves to prevent later disturbance of the child-caregiver relationship. This protective effect is observed in the sample as a whole, however it is even stronger for first admissions. Furthermore, it appears that disease category is relevant for the risk of psychological disturbance, as it is for hospitalization history. The long-term effect of hospitalization on behavior problems is expressed as an effect size according to the model of Cohen (1977). It is rather small in the entire sample, but marked in the condition of insufficient parental attendance. In the next and final chapter the findings are integrated and interpreted, after an extensive discussion of validity.

CHAPTER 7 DISCUSSION AND CONCLUSIONS

This chapter is devoted to the results of the research project. Final conclusions must be preceded by discussions of validity. In Section 7.1 any possible validity problems of the prospective study will be critically reviewed; one unforeseen problem will be scrutinized. In Section 7.2 conclusions will be drawn pertaining to the eleven hypotheses that were initially presented in Section 3.1. A theoretical interpretation of the findings in terms of underlying processes is attempted in Section 7.3. Finally a modest program of recommendations for prevention is offered in Section 7.4.

7.1   Validity

Drawing upon the well known treatment of validity problems by Cook and Campbell (1979) four aspects of validity should be distinguished: statistical conclusion validity, internal validity, external validity, and construct validity. Each of these four aspects will be evaluated, and a number of strong and weak points of the present study will be illuminated.

Statistical conclusion validity

The expected rate of type I errors in our analysis is related to the choice: alpha = .05, for each of the many F-tests required to reach a verdict on eleven hypotheses. If every implied null-hypothesis had been true, and the actual error-proportion had been 5%, 2 of the 41 values of F, reported in Chapter 5 would have been (erroneously) significant. The actual number of significant values was 11, excluding unpredicted findings, which does not seem to be a chance result. Some doubt may have been raised, however, by the apparent selection of 'successful' dependent variables. The variables *disturbance of relationship* and BSQ_3 were post hoc identified as the most sensitive and valid criteria. This was implicit in the testing of four hypotheses: Hypotheses 5, 6, 7, and 8. Although the objection is a valid reason for special caution, the statistical conclusion validity of these four hypotheses is not really affected. Hypotheses 5, 7 and 8 are disconfirmed. The one hypothesis that was counted as having been confirmed, in spite of negative results with several dependent variables, is Hypothesis 6, which predicted the beneficial effects of parental presence. If confirmation of this crucial hypothesis had been based on an isolated statistic, it could have been a chance result. Evidence for Hypothesis 6, however, was found in Tables 5.8, 5.10, 5.12, 5.13, and Appendix 3.2. This may be called a robust effect. In a survey of results, it may be concluded that the threat of type I errors has been sufficiently restricted.

Random heterogeneity of respondents is listed as a threat to statistical validity, while homogeneity of respondents is mentioned as a threat to external validity (Cook & Campbell, 1979). Our study embodies a compromise between the two. A great number of variables can influence the central concept, adjustment of the infant, for example socioeconomic status, belonging to an ethnic minority, perinatal problems and so on. Some of these factors are recorded, but none was used for selection. The effect of heterogeneity is random variance, that must be included as error variance in the testing of various hypothetical relations. The danger is not a type I error but a type II error. Some of our hypotheses, for instance Hypothesis 1, 5 and 8, might have been supported if the sample had been either much larger, or more homogeneous on some conventional criterion. This latter condition, however, would exclude subjects included in the theory and constitute a disadvantage to the relevance of positive findings.

Internal validity

A number of factors, such as history and maturation may act as threats to internal validity if they interact with (the assignment of) treatment. This is relevant for our experimental set-up, where cases were assigned to the experimental group when the consultant was available. In many cases such assignment was dependent purely on the moment of entry; the order in which new cases were identified. This is true for completely planned admissions that constitute 86% of the sample. In nine cases the date of admission was the first available opportunity to visit the family: six were emergency admissions and three were admissions that had been rescheduled or fixed at the last possible moment. Among this group only two interventions were done, because of insufficient opportunity. This category may bias the comparison of experimentals and controls. In order to check this effect, the nine special cases were compared to the rest of the sample on three principal variables: BSQ_1, BSQ_3, and parental presence. A t-test yielded insignificant differences, with p-values (two-sided) larger than .60. Although such a check is not foolproof, the likelihood that a hypothesis is falsely rejected or accepted because of this source of error seems to be small.

Two hospitals contributed five cases, but none of them were included in the experimental group. This circumstance is a similar cause of possible bias. However, when a comparison was made between experimentals and controls excluding these five cases a significant difference was still found; therefore the initial finding remains valid.

The experimental group was found to be somewhat, albeit slightly, at a disadvantage for preadmission adjustment and previous admissions. Because preadmission adjustment is a strong predictor of later adjustment this may introduce bias. We hope there has been effective adjustment for such bias in the analysis.

An entirely different danger, that might cause a type II error, is the possibility that the control group has been unintentionally influenced by the same, or a similar treatment effect which enhanced parental presence for experimentals. Diffusion of treatment is transmission of treatment effect to controls, for example by communication between subjects from these two groups. The latter has incidentally occurred, but such contacts have been sufficiently rare to dismiss their influence. Much more likely is the possibility that parents in the control group have been alerted to the psychological risks of hospitalization by the fact of their participation in the research project, particularly by answering questions about the adjustment of their infants. Such a mechanism may have increased parental presence among controls, and therefore an underestimation of the effects of interventions.

External validity

The issue of external validity concerns the validity of conclusion for different settings and different patients from the same or a similar population. There are several reasons for confidence about external validity. The conclusions are certainly not limited to a specific setting or specific category of disease, a limitation of many related investigations. While six hospitals have contributed, it should be noted that the hospitals are not chosen at random: university hospitals have provided 70% of the sample, simply because university hospitals are more apt than other hospitals for many problems requiring major surgery. An important characteristic of participating hospitals is that parental presence was not severely restricted by hospital rules. As explained in Section 1.3 other hospitals might have more restrictions on parental presence during induction of anaesthesia. Presumably the findings reported here can be generalized to any up-to-date Dutch hospital where major surgery on children is practiced. Attachment-theoretical principles that were confirmed by this study are not restricted to any specific setting.

The external validity of the study is certainly restricted to children of the age range studied: this restriction is explicit in the theoretical framework. We can be fairly confident that the results may be generalized to the population studied, because selection and attrition effects have been decidedly low (compare Table 3.1). The number of refusals is about the minimum that might have been expected. The high degree of participation should be explained by the conviction of parents, frequently expressed, that research of this kind can contribute to reduction of developmental risk for some toddlers. Whether the conclusions are valid for non-surgical pediatric patients with similar hospitalization experience is a matter of speculation.

Construct validity

The constructs we have measured are valid if they truly represent the concepts that figure as causes and effects in our theory. For some measurements this will be granted without further scrutiny. Special discussion may be devoted to attachment quality, disturbance of relationship and the measurements of general adjustment: PHBQ, BSQ and ego-resilience.

The concept of attachment quality is so thoroughly linked with the Strange Situation that the validity of any new procedure is most readily conceived as concurrent validity: degree of agreement with the traditional procedure. This criterion could not be applied.

Confidence in the present measure of attachment quality is mainly based on the theoretical framework of the Strange Situation and the similarity of the situation created in the hospital environment. If the theory in which the Strange Situation is embedded remains valid when tested in a different but related situation, then the present assessments of attachment quality are also valid. An additional point to be made is that these assessments were produced by experts in attachment theory, fully trained in the traditional method. A reasonable, although not very strong, agreement was observed in a test series without adjustment or specification of conventional methods (Section 4.4). To sum up: empirical confirmation of the attachment quality classifications is actually weak, nevertheless there are reasons to have faith in them and no strong reason to distrust them.

Disturbance of the relationship between infant and caregiver, perhaps a transient phenomenon, was obtained by adding the scores for avoidance and negativity. These constructs were conceived and made operational by Erickson et al. (1985), who found that avoidance discriminated significantly between securely attached children with behavior problems and securely attached children without behavior problems ($t = -2.90$; $p = .01$). Negativity had a similar effect, which, however, was not significant ($t = -.151$; $p = .17$). The findings of Erickson et al. were to a certain extent replicated. Taking BSQ_2 as the measure of behavior problems we found $t = -.90$ ($p = .19$) for avoidance and $t = -1.37$ ($p = .10$) for negativity, among securely attached children. Moreover, the correlations of avoidance and negativity with BSQ_2 in the whole sample were only .07 and .18. On the other hand, the relationship of these measures to parental presence in hospital can not be attributed to any common source of error, because the scores are obtained on different occasions with different methods, by different observers. Moreover, although disturbance of relationship was not predictive of behavioral problems

(BSQ$_3$) it did predict delayed language development.

In interpreting results we have been baffled by two unexpected findings: (1) the fact that PHBQ-scores, which represented posthospital maladjustment, were *lower* in the case of low parental presence and in the case of membership of the control group; (2) the fact that BSQ-scores at t_2 were unrelated to parental presence, while at t_3 they were related as predicted. These results were obtained despite all the data documenting the reliability and validity of the two instruments, both from previous research and from the present study.

In the case of the PHBQ it was initially suspected that the revision of the scale, to adapt it to our population, might have been the cause of trouble. This explanation, however, could be ruled out by computing separate subscores from original items and from new items. It was found that a scale of exclusively original items had the same tendency.

A different explanation suggested that post-hospital behavior may have been truly different from what had been expected from the literature: children could perhaps become more demanding ('spoiled') by parental support, or conversely, in the case of low parental support, develop avoidant behavior which might be scored as reflecting a lower degree of maladjustment. To demonstrate the inadequacy of this interpretation we list four behaviors reported to have been comparatively frequent in the case of higher levels of parental attendance in hospital:
- increase in fits of anger (PHBQ 18)
- increase in sleeping with parents (PHBQ 4)
- more demanding of parent (PHBQ 25)
- increase of attention seeking (PHBQ 21)

Although it is conceivable that such behaviors are increased by parental presence in hospital, this is unlikely for all for of them, and hardly compatible with the observed *prevention* of disturbance in the relationship. Moreover, it was found that three of these behaviors (items 18, 4 and 21) are significantly reduced at t_3 if parental presence is sufficient. This was demonstrated in Section 6.3, by analyzing BSQ-topics that refer to exactly the same behaviors. If the PHBQ-scores had been true, this specific decrease was preceded by a specific increase, which is not very likely.

The most fitting explanation is that the unexpected findings represent a response tendency of parents fostered by uncertainty about the adequacy of their participation in hospital. Particularly susceptible to this influence would be the parent-report measures that were taken early after discharge: PHBQ and BSQ$_2$. The PHBQ is the more susceptible because the questions relate to pre-post change of behavior in children. These changes may be hard to judge, unless they are obvious. Some mothers had a tendency to proclaim the behavior of their child unchanged by any criterion. Presumably this tendency was stronger for mothers in the control group, who had not been invited to discuss their worries. They may have given answers that were influenced by wishful thinking without being aware of it. Unfortunately there is no way of checking this explanation.

The explanation does take account of the anomalous findings with BSQ$_2$ as well as with the PHBQ. The BSQ$_2$-scores may represent a compound of true posthospitalization disturbance and opposed response tendencies. *Observations* such as the ratings for avoidance and negativity could not be affected by this factor.

A word should be devoted to ego-resiliency. The scores for ego-resiliency proved to be related to BSQ$_3$-scores and do not produce anomalous results. They were apparently less strongly related to the process variables because some subjects were too young for this instrument. The instrument *can* be used for children of 30 months or even younger (a quarter of the sample at t_3), but it is not really suitable for this age category.

7.2   Survey of results from the prospective study

Non-supported hypotheses

The notion was refuted that posthospital maladjustment would be more likely if attachment is insecure. Even very recently it has been suggested (de Boer, 1992) that secure attachment should be considered a protective factor during hospitalization. Such was implied in the hypothesis. Judging by our data, however, securely attached infants have at least as much need of their parent during stress as those classified as insecurely attached and will show posthospital maladjustment if insufficiently supported.

The expectation, or rather the hope, that the increase in parental involvement achieved by interventions would be reflected in better adjustment scores of the toddler, was also unconfirmed. In fact, all posthospital adjustment scores of the experimental group except disturbance of the relationship were unfavorable, when compared to the control group. To be sure, a slight disadvantage was recorded at the outset. The gain in parental attendance achieved by interventions is not very large. In the case of a family where the parents are adequately involved without additional encouragement an increase of presence (due to intervention) may not contribute much to prevention of subsequent problems.

The finding that duration of admission was not significantly related to posthospital maladjustment suggests that the influence of duration is smaller than we tend to think. Both the research literature and common sense indicate that long hospitalization in early childhood is deleterious in comparison to admissions restricted to a few days. The range of duration in our sample does not include these extremes. Apparently the difference between one week or three weeks in hospital does not strongly affect adjustment.

Maladjustment was predictable from hospitalization history, but at t_1 , before the prospectively studied admission, the effect was not significant. A plausible interpretation would be that many children at t_1 have recovered from the effects of their first or second admission. After renewed admission, however, negative effects of hospitalization history become visible. It is apparent from the data that the record has implications for adjustment at t_2 and t_3.

Hypotheses that were supported

Adequate preadmission adjustment, despite previous hospital experience, indicates decreased or low vulnerability, in the sense that a new admission may be sustained without serious damage. This can be explained by the fact that the subject has found that he/she can cope with such experiences, presumably accompanied by an attachment figure. The finding may contribute to an assessment of the situation at the time of admission. Moreover, it has some theoretical significance in connection with the concept of stress-inoculation advocated by Damsté (1981).

Interventions directed towards the parents can effect better parental support. This result is confirmed by experimental standards. It is true that the increase in parental support was found to be modest. As explained in the discussion of internal validity, the effect of interventions may have been underestimated, because of a potentially similar effect among controls by the mere process of measurement.

The finding that quality of posthospital adjustment is related to parental support in hospital is of vital importance, although for some people this may represent a truism. Availability of parents and support during the hospital episode proved to be a better predictor of long-term adjustment than sensitivity, although sensitivity was a strong predictor of language development. The two dimensions of parental support apparently reflect a great deal of the environment of the toddler and its potential to foster psychosocial development, in spite of illness.

Evidence was obtained that the relationship between child and parent may be affected by hospital treatment if parental attendance is insufficient. In Chapter 1 this was theoretically explained and three studies were cited to provide support for the proposition that avoidant attachment may be produced by hospital experience. In the present sample 30% avoidant attachments were found, a figure larger than the standard, perhaps because of previous hospitalization experience. Finally, two months after discharge, avoidance and negativity toward the parent during a play-session were found to have increased in children where parental presence in hospital had been comparatively low.

This survey of results can be concluded with findings on language acquisition. As has been mentioned, sensitivity proved to be a strong predictor of the development of language comprehension and language expression. Parental presence in hospital did not predict this development. However, an interactional effect of the number of hospital admissions and the degree of parental attendance revealed that language acquisition was delayed if both factors were unfavorable. Disturbance of the relationship between toddler and parent was demonstrated as impairing the growth of language comprehension.

7.3   Underlying processes

The nature of disturbances after early hospitalization

Besides specific results, fruits of hypothesis testing and exploratory analysis, we hope to acquire a general understanding of the process of emotional response to the hospitalization experience. This should be attempted by an integration of the new findings and inclusion of results accumulated by others. A certain amount of speculation is indispensable. The first general question is whether the adverse effects of hospitalization can be conceived of as disruption of attachment security. We think this interpretation is now supported by several facts.

Firstly we recall the distribution of attachment quality found in Strange Situation investigations of infants with a hospitalization history, data that were described in Section 1.3.
It emerged that about 40% avoidant attachments were observed in this population, where 20% is normative amongst non-hospitalized subjects. The data of Ainsworth et al. (1978) collected during home observation of avoidantly attached children, imply that *anger toward the parent* is specifically characteristic of this category of children. Although *within the Strange Situation* expressions of anger are more common in the case of ambivalent, type C attachment, this is explained by inhibition on the part of avoidant children. The correlation of the secure/avoidant distinction (represented by the discriminant function) with expressions of anger at home was no less than .79.

Secondly, important clues are to be found in the experimental results of Hoeksma and Koomen (1991). They observed a substantial increase of avoidant behavior on the part of the child towards the mother after hospitalization, both during Strange Situations staged in the laboratory, and during interactions after a more or less stressful separation in the home. They interpret this unmistakable effect as a simultaneous activation of both attachment behavior and anger. In the course of a period of three to six months afterwards, in which no readmission occurred, the effect seemed to subside.

Thirdly, in our own prospective study, we observed avoidant behavior towards the parent in non-stressful play episodes in the home, two months after hospitalization. Scores for avoidance in the sense of withdrawal from interaction with the parent appeared to be strongly correlated with scores for negativity, the expression of anger, dislike, or hostility towards the parent, assigned to the same interactions. The degree of such behavior was inversely related to independent (in the sense of non-contaminated) scores for parental attendance in the hospital. Moreover, for patients without a hospitalization history at the start, this avoidant and angry behavior in the early follow-up was a foreboding of relational behavior problems such as attention seeking and noncompliance during later development (r=.42 ; p<.05). In the sample as a whole, avoidance and negativity predicted a slower development of language comprehension.

Our interpretation is that, for the at-risk population of young patients considered here, damage to the security of attachment after hospitalization is not a rare occurrence. If this picture is correct, the relational disturbances observed in the prospective study represent disturbances of attachment quality, linked with feelings of anger towards the attachment figure. The disruption of security may of course be open to recovery, as suggested by the Hoeksma & Koomen (1991) data.

In the theoretical review presented in Chapter 1 the concept of stress was emphasized. Absence of the attachment figure at critical moments was identified as a an important contribution to stressful and potentially traumatic experience. In retrospect it seems a possibility that disruption of secure attachment in itself is sufficient explanation of subsequent maladjustment. This can not be decided at present with any certainty. The fact that the sheer amount of hospital experience is a predictor of long term problems, as found in the retrospective study, complicates the picture. In our final speculations we will consider factors that may help to explain the relational disturbance.

Preconditions of relational disturbance

If the child's anger toward the parent is regarded as a principal factor in disturbed attachment, the origin of this anger should be carefully considered. First, as emphasized before, not the events in the hospital as such, but the meanings of these events for the child need to be understood. It may be attempted to explain the anger of children after surgery by the fact of their cognitive immaturity.

Whereas the prospective study confirmed the importance of parental attendance, the retrospective study suggested that surgery and pain contributed to the development of behavior problems. This certainly contradicts the viewpoint that problems might be reduced to the strangeness of the hospital environment and the separation from parents. The behavior problems that were implicated, like attention seeking and soiling, may be considered as possible symptoms of attachment insecurity, even if insufficient as diagnostic criteria. The question is whether blaming the parent for anxiety, pain and discomfort is a plausble response on the part of the child.

Adults are apt both to underestimate and overestimate the cognitive faculties of two-year-olds. A recent trend in developmental psychology calls attention to the development of metacognition (Flavell, 1979), a concept referring to knowledge about cognition itself, for example being aware that a specific impression may be either valid or deceptive, and the regulation of cognition, for example checking for error. It has been demonstrated that the so-called appearance-reality distinction, a form of metacognition where a distinction is made between true properties of a physical object and its appearance to the subject, *can not be learned* until the age of three or four (Flavell, Green & Flavell, 1986).

It is desirable that an infant going to hospital comprehends, at least in an inarticulate fashion, that what happens is for its own wellbeing. Even infants are supposed to make some distinction between medical treatment and maltreatment, an experience that is apparently conducive to avoidant attachment, according to the meta-analysis of Van IJzendoorn et al.

(1991). *In fact this distinction may be beyond the cognitive potential of an eighteen month old infant.*

Main (1991) has suggested that it is precisely the lack of metacognitive control and ensuing immature cognitions of infants which makes them vulnerable to disruption of secure attachment. Her hypothesis is that some conditions provoke the creation of multiple, incompatible working models of attachment figures, for example the supportive parent versus the malignant parent. This hypothetical mental process certainly involves a serious disruption of affective bonds. The idea may seem plausible, considering circumstantial evidence, but it is at present highly speculative.

In some cases the child may experience the treatment as punishment, a tendency that was repeatedly found in five-year-olds, as related in Section 1.1. The specific cognitive and emotional processes are not directly accessible, and moreover will depend on the individual infant. The statement that parents are sometimes blamed for the considerable stress of medical treatment, however, is not just a conjecture. In several cases unmistakable expressions of anger and rejection after surgery were spontaneously reported by parents.

If age-dependent cognitive distortions are a factor contributing to disturbance of the relationship, the association of age at the time of admission with disturbance of relationship may be revealing. It was examined in the sample of the prospective study. An inverted U-shape was found, with the highest incidence of disturbance in the 15-20 months age range. This exploratory result is certainly compatible with the hypotheses discussed above.

In the traditional account of attachment the risk of disturbance caused by separations is emphasized. If the final explanations offered here are correct, events other than separation, such as pain and fear may have a similar impact. Nevertheless, lack of parental presence was clearly identified as a factor contributing to disturbance of the relationship, despite the daily care provided even in the 'low' condition of parental presence.

7.4   Recommendations

Considering the results reported with a view to practical consequences, three findings can be emphasized.

(1) It is established that parental participation as a phenomenon has been increasing steadily during the past ten years. According to our data, parental participation has been sufficiently practiced by about 60% of families, *without* intervention. (As explained in Section 7.1 this estimate may be inflated.) The *growth* of parental involvement can be seen as a reinforcement of current policy.

(2) Although several theoretical principles of the present study were confirmed, the efficacy of interventions to prevent maladjustment could not be demonstrated.

(3) Some symptoms of long-term disturbance of socio-emotional development were clearly associated with insufficient parental attendance. In the clinical setting such insufficiency of parental attendance is not usually recognized, unless it is *gross* insufficiency.

The outcomes (2) and (3) can be theoretically reconciled. This may be difficult where the validity of recommendations is an issue. Those who wish to emphasize (2) will not really be interested in outcome (3) and have no need of further reform. Those who wish to emphasize (3) may conclude, despite (2), that prevention is still possible and that additional encouragement of parental attendance is called for. The latter stance implies that the policy of the staff should be to take responsibility for parental attendance beyond the mere provision of facilities. Only from this viewpoint can any recommendation be valued. Recommendations then should be guided by theory and previously accumulated knowledge, as well as by the present findings.

The guideline for prevention of posthospital maladjustment proposed here embodies the following principles:

- it is intended for a specific age range;
- it is based on a concept of non-medical risk that can be assessed by the hospital staff;
- it is aimed at parents, in the assumption that parental participation will prevent problems;
- it recognizes the autonomy of parents, as well as the idea that they frequently need information and/or support.

The first of these principles is based on the literature, the second and third partly on the literature, partly on the results of the present study. The fourth principle is only based on knowledge of current clinical practice. Before elaborating on these principles the essential references are summarized:

The relevance of age (Sections 1.1 and 1.3) is validated by the literature. The decline of risk with age is found by Prugh et al. (1953), Vernon et al. (1966), Brain & Maclay (1968), Douglas (1975), and Mrazek (1984). The increase of risk during the first year of life has been meticulously observed and described by Schaffer and Callender (1959). The general conclusions concerning age are endorsed by the major reviews of Vernon et al. (1965) and Thompson (1985). Evidence that very short admissions are comparatively harmless, judged by short-term follow-up, has been obtained by Davenport and Werry (1970). This result was confirmed by a recent unpublished study in the Netherlands by Meursing (personal communication). Evidence for the extra risk of multiple hospital admissions is found in Douglas (1975), Quinton & Rutter (1976), and in the present study: Sections 5.3 and 7.2. The influence of preadmission emotional adjustment was found by Brain & Maclay (1968) and Dearden (1970). It was confirmed in the present study (Section 5.3).

A specific age range

The research reported was limited to the age range of 12-36 months. This age range was selected for many reasons, discussed in Sections 1.1 and 1.3. Children over 36 months become progressively more open to explanation and perhaps less vulnerable to disruptions of attachment.

Hospitalization may be a threat, for example, to a child of 5 months, a child of 24 months and a child of 48 months. Because of the developmental stage, however, the threat is different in each case. The difference is not simply a difference of degree. For the younger or older child a different protocol may be suitable, but this decision is outside the scope of the present discussion.

Of course it would not be wise to pretend that a developmental stage could be sharply demarcated by age boundaries. For a childrens' ward the practical question would be whether all children being tended could be considered as being of one developmental stage. To be pragmatic, this may be presumed, if, for example, all patients are in the range of 6-30 months, or in the age range of 20-42 months, but not if the range is 12-60 months. If the age range is wide, a distinction between younger and older patients may be useful and 36 months is proposed as a boundary. For those under 6 months a different protocol may be appropriate. The age difference is emphasized to clarify the nature and the degree of risk. It is not intended to suggest any restrictions for parents with children outside the critical range.

A conception of non-medical risk

The conception of *medical* risk in the case of surgical intervention is familiar. Assessment of medical risk is considered necessary although sometimes difficult. It is proposed here that assessment of the *non-medical* risk of posthospital maladjustment is equally important and perhaps easier.

When an admission is planned with parents, a conception of non-medical risk should be available. This should be of a very simple nature. Four criteria of non-medical risk can be applied. The *first* is age, which has already been discussed. The *second* is duration. It has been found that a short admission of one or two days, including surgery, need not be a serious threat to posthospital adjustment. The *third* criterion is the number of previous admissions. It was found in our data that previous admissions could not significantly predict preadmission adjustment, but the number of previous admissions could predict posthospital adjustment and is therefore an indicator of vulnerability: latent vulnerability. This is one aspect of non-medical risk, that should be discussed with parents. The *fourth* criterion is the preadmission adjustment of the infant, reported by the caregiver. This was found to be a valid predictor among infants with an extended hospitalization history. An assessment of prehospital adjustment may be done formally, with the help of an instrument, like the behavior problem scale of the BSQ, which should take 20-30 minutes. But such a formal approach is not mandatory. For a clinician it may be sufficient to explore posthospital behavior after previous admissions and current behaviors like sleeping and eating.

For clinical purposes a scale of risk might be constructed. At present, however, it would be a considerable improvement if each criterion of risk were to be systematically taken into account. No computation is needed.

The assumption that parental participation will prevent problems

The attachment theory seems to provide the most promising ideas for prevention. Forms of parental participation that can be recommended are:
- presence of at least one parent during most of the daytime, including parental responsibility for non-medical care;
- presence and involvement of a parent during routine measurements (body temperature), injections or similar invasions of the body, and examinations;
- rooming-in, which is entirely different from spending the night elsewhere in the hospital or in guest rooms;
- presence during induction of anaesthesia.

These options are recommended in any case, but most urgently when the degree of non-medical risk is judged to be comparatively high. The question whether obstacles are found against practice of such participation in an individual case, and what, if anything, can be done to overcome such obstacles, should be discussed with parents of patients if the admission is to last several days. If the hospitalization is planned a discussion with parents should be arranged before the day of actual admission. It might be part of the consultation where a decision about treatment is taken. Solutions for insufficient knowledge and practical problems of parents will be too late when the situation is discussed at the time of admission, or even later. Practical problems should be anticipated. A new video-program for the specific purpose of introducing inexperienced parents to the possibilities and problems of their participation in hospital has recently become available (Uitvlugt, 1992).

The autonomy of parents and their need of information and support

The autonomy of parents, where participation in hospital is concerned, is frequently emphasized by the hospital staff. Of course parents can not be forced to participate. Nor is moral pressure acceptable, or even useful, when parents decline the opportunity to be present support their infant. The attitudes of parents should be respected and some circumstances may prohibit their attendance in hospital. On the other hand, just asking parents whether they have planned to be present, for instance if they have decided to make use of opportunities for rooming-in, neglects the fact that many people are not aware of the serious consequences that such a decision may entail. It is essential that parents should be informed about the specific risks of their absence, even when obstacles exist that cannot be removed by timely consultation or planning.

Nurses and pedagogical co-workers are apprehensive of intrusions upon the private situations and decisions of parents. This is no problem at all when parents are prepared to participate anyway, but for the reasons stated above it may be a problem when parents do not appreciate the value of their presence in hospital. Therefore the person who is selected to discuss these matters should be sufficiently experienced and understanding. Her or his ability to establish rapport with parents, to respect their ideas, and still to provide a good picture of the interests of infants in this situation is the crux of any attempt at prevention.

To sum up, and conclude our recommendations:

(1)   The notion of psychological risk has obtained a firmer foundation in research. Four criteria have been identified for practical application.

(2)   Reasons have been advanced to cultivate parental participation, for example rooming-in, for any small patient with a special non-medical risk factor.

(3)   Practical problems of hospitals and parents in the execution of this program should be studied.

SUMMARY

The first chapter is concerned with past research and theoretical ideas. It has been established that the socio-emotional development of young infants may be affected by hospital treatment, depending on a number of conditions. For the majority of children in hospital no severe problems are to be expected, because they are no longer of the most sensitive age, not staying more than one or a few days, not readmitted at an early age, not severely hurt or restricted in freedom by treatment, and/or not left without parental support for a substantial amount of time. If circumstances are not favorable psychological disturbances may be apparent after discharge, especially in the 6-36 months age range.

British studies of long-term effects have suggested that, if adverse conditions prevail, emotional scars may remain for any number of years. These studies are presumably outdated as regards the incidence of such unfavorable conditions, especially the absence of attachment figures in the hospital. It must be admitted however, that the effects of present day policy for patients who are at risk is unknown.

For a theoretical explanation it is proposed here that hospital experience may become traumatic if the degree of stress in the hospital situation is felt to be beyond any available coping mechanism. It may sooner be experienced as such when attachment figures, usually parents, are inaccessible. On the other hand, if the situation is found to be manageable the tolerance for future admissions may become enhanced. Initial secure attachment is hypothesized to be a protective factor. The hypothesis is discussed that the hospitalization experience may entail damage to the quality of the attachment relationship between child and caregiver. In particular it may occur that secure attachment gives way to avoidant attachment. This idea is supported by data of three empirical studies into attachment quality of chronically ill infants and their mothers. The crucial protection seems to be parental support during the hospital experience, as is suggested and supported by research on the preventive value of rooming-in. This support factor can be distinguished into parental sensitivity and parental attendance.

The conditions that are presumed important here have been investigated and tested in two studies that are the substance of this book. The first is a small-sample retrospective study, comprised by Chapter 2. Here behavioral disturbance of children with hospitalization history is studied about three years after the latest discharge. It is compared with controls of the same mean age. The most important general conclusion of the study is that adverse effects of hospitalization may persist for years if conditions are unfavorable, as they are for a minority of children. The results confirm the relevance of prevention. To explore possibilities for prevention a different research project is designed: the larger and more complicated prospective study.

The prospective study involves 64 surgical patients and their families. The research design, described in Chapter 3, quantifies several aspects of child-caregiver interactions, before, during and after hospitalization of the child. Patients are selected by age (12-36 months) and the necessity of surgery which requires a hospital stay of at least seven days. Parental support in hospital is the central theme. The last follow-up is scheduled at a time that implies complete recovery from temporary upset. The dependent variables include parental report of posthospital behavior symptoms, observation of child-caregiver interactions and language development. Interventions are designed to promote parental support in a part of the sample. Eleven hypotheses are formulated on the effect of various conditions that may influence post-hospital disturbance.

Chapter 4 serves to describe the sample and the observed degree of parental participation

in the hospital. Moreover, the many instruments and scales are examined and improved by psychometric techniques. An analysis and description of the sample yields a large variety of medical (surgical) problems, as has been intended. Instruments and scales are employed in order to measure the following constructs:
- hospitalization history
- preadmission adjustment / behavior problems
- parental sensitivity (video-obsevation)
- initial attachment security (video-observation)
- parental attendance in hospital
- short-term upset after discharge
- behavior problems (maladjustment) during follow-up
- disturbance of relationship to caregiver (video-observation)
- ego-resilience
- language development

The analysis and results are described in Chapter 5.

A number of expected and unexpected results were obtained. Maladjustment was predictable from *hospitalization history*, (hypothesis 1), but at t_1 , before the prospectively studied admission, the effect was not significant. After renewed admission, however, negative effects of hospitalization history become visible. It is apparent from the data that the record has implications for adjustment at t_2 , two months after dicharge and at t_3 , at least nine months after discharge.

Hypothesis (2), suggesting that vulnerability might be gauged by a combination of data on previous hospitalizations and preadmission adjustment, was supported. If the latter is clearly satifactory the non-medical risk is less.

An effect of interventions on parental presence, predicted by hypothesis (3), was confirmed. However, indirect effects of interventions on posthospital adjustment of the child, predicted by hypothesis (4) were not found.

Hypothesis (5) presumed that posthospital adjustment would be related to duration of the hospital episode; it was disconfirmed for the range of durations examined here. Posthospital adjustment was related to parental support as predicted by hypothesis (6). Significant effects were obtained at t_2 for disturbance of relationship and at t_3 for reported behavior problems. Of the two aspects of parental support: sensitivity and presence in hospital, only the latter was found to be a significant predictor of general adjustment at the time of late follow-up. Sensitivity, on the other hand, did predict the development of language acquisition.

In Hypothesis (7) secure attachment was conjectured to be a protective factor. This was not substantiated: subsequent adjustment of initially securely attached infants was average in the case of sufficient parental presence, but severely damaged if parental presence was comparatively low. An interactional effect of duration and parental presence, as specified in hypothesis (8), was not confirmed. Parental presence did influence disturbance of relationship, however: insufficient parental presence enhanced avoidant behavior, as suggested in hypothesis (9).

Hypothesis (11), concerning effects of the hospital episode on language development, was to a large extent confirmed. An interactional effect of hospitalization history and (lack of) parental attendance in hospital on language acquisition was found. Furthermore, scores of 'disturbed relationship' were strongly related to language comprehension, but sensitivity was the best predictor of language development, both of comprehension and of expression.

From additional analyses in Chapter 6 it may be concluded that rooming-in serves to prevent later disturbance of the child-caregiver relationship. This protective effect is observed in the sample as a whole, moreover it is even stronger for first admissions. In the same chapter patients with different diseases are compared. It appears that disease category is relevant for the risk of psychological disturbance, a difference which may be mediated by hospitalization history. The long-term effect of hospitalization on behavior problems is expressed as an effect size according to the model of Cohen (1977). It is rather small in the entire sample, but marked in the condition of insufficient parental attendance.

A basic result is the evidence that the relationship between child and parent may be affected by hospital treatment if parental attendance is insufficient. Two months after discharge, avoidance and negativity toward the parent during a play-session were found to have increased in children where parental presence in hospital had been comparatively low.

In the first section of Chapter 7 the validity of the prospective study is critically reviewed. One weakness is the possibility that parental care has been enhanced in the control group by participation in the research and answering pretest questionnaires. Furthermore reasons are found to distrust the parent-report measures obtained shortly after discharge; they seem to be fraught with bias that is absent in the observational measures.

Our interpretation of the findings suggests that, for the at-risk population of young patients considered here, damage to the security of attachment after hospitalization is not a rare occurrence. An increase of avoidant attachment is likely. If this inference is correct, the relational disturbances observed in the prospective study represent disturbances of attachment quality, linked with feelings of anger towards the attachment figure(s). This phenomenon may be understood better if the cognitive immaturity of the very young is taken into account; it is possible that parents are in some way blamed for the pain and anxiety of the treatment as well as for intermittent absence. In the final section of the last chapter some possible guidelines for prevention are formulated.

(a)   prevention should be intended for a specific age range;
(b)   it should be based on a concept of non-medical risk that can be assessed by the hospital staff;
(c)   it must be aimed at parents, in the assumption that parental participation will prevent problems;
(d)   it recognizes the autonomy of parents, as well as the idea that they frequently need information and/or support.

Four criteria can be considered for risk-assessment of an impending hospitalization episode:
1.   *age: 6 - 36 months*
2.   *duration: expected number of nights more than two?*
3.   *hospitalization history*
4.   *general adjustment before admission*

It is urged that the *planning* of an admission in the specified age range should include a discussion of non-medical risk and of the possible prevention by parental attendance.

SAMENVATTING

Het eerste hoofdstuk betreft voorafgaand onderzoek over de psychologische gevolgen van ziekenhuisverblijf en theoretische uitgangspunten. Vastgesteld is dat de socio-emotionele ontwikkeling van jonge kinderen door een ziekenhuisopname ongunstig kan worden beinvloed, afhankelijk van de omstandigheden waaronder de opname plaatsvindt. Voor de meerderheid van kinderen die opgenomen worden zijn geen langdurige problemen te verwachten, omdat ze niet in de meest kwetsbare leeftijdsfase verkeren, niet meer dan enkele dagen in het ziekenhuis verblijven, niet op korte termijn heropgenoemen worden, niet heel veel pijn of vrijheidsbeperkingen ondergaan en/of niet lang van ouderlijke ondersteuning verstoken blijven. Als de combinatie van omstandigheden ongunstig is worden menigmaal nadelige effecten waargenomen, vooral in de leeftijd tussen 6 en 36 maanden.

Britse studies over de gevolgen van ziekenhuisopname op langere termijn hebben de indruk gewekt dat, indien de situatie ongunstig is, emotionele beschadigingen de ontwikkeling jarenlang kunnen beinvloeden. Deze onderzoekingen zijn vermoedelijk verouderd wat betreft de frequentie waarmee ongunstige omstandigheden, met name de afwezigheid van gehechtheidsfiguren, zich voordoen. Het blijft echter een probleem dat de resultaten van het hedendaags beleid voor risico-groepen onvoldoende zijn onderzocht.

De theoretische verklaring die hier wordt voorgesteld houdt in dat een ziekenhuiservaring traumatische gevolgen kan hebben als de mate van stress onbeheersbaar is voor de beschikbare *coping-mechanismen*. Deze situatie zou zich eerder kunnen voordoen gedurende de tijden dat gehechtheidsfiguren, gewoonlijk de ouders, niet beschikbaar zijn. Anderzijds, als de stress van de ziekenhuisopname hanteerbaar blijkt, zou de tolerantie voor toekomstige ziekenhuiservaringen kunnen toenemen. Veilige gehechtheid kan hypothetisch worden beschouwd als een beschermende factor. Daarnaast moet de hypothese worden overwogen dat ziekenhuiservaringen schade kunnen veroorzaken aan de kwaliteit van de gehechtheidsrelatie. Meer in het bijzonder zou veilige gehechtheid kunnen veranderen in vermijdende gehechtheid. Een drietal onderzoekingen naar de gehechtheidskwaliteit in de relatie tussen chronisch zieke kinderen en hun ouders wijst in deze richting. Een kritieke factor in het proces is wellicht de mate van steun die het kind ondervindt van de kant van de ouders tijdens de opname. Deze veronderstelling, in de lijn van het voorgaande, wordt krachtig gesteund door een aantal onderzoekingen naar de preventieve waarde van rooming-in. Het is echter van belang onderscheid te maken tussen twee aspecten van de manier waarop ouders het kind steunen: sensitiviteit in de omgang met het kind en aanwezigheid in het ziekenhuis.

De oorzakelijke factoren waaraan in deze zienswijze een belangrijke rol wordt toegekend zijn het onderwerp van een tweetal onderzoekingen die in dit boek worden gerapporteerd. De eerste is een retrospectieve studie van beperkte omvang, die geheel in hoofdstuk 2 wordt beschreven. Gedragsproblemen van kinderen met een opname-geschiedenis worden circa drie jaar na ontslag bestudeerd. Er wordt een vergelijking gemaakt met kinderen in dezelfde leeftijdsfase zonder opnamegeschiedenis. De belangrijkste algemene conclusie is dat nadelige gevolgen van ziekenhuisverblijf gedurende ettelijke jaren nadien de ontwikkeling van het kind kunnen beinvloeden. De uitkomsten onderstrepen het belang van pogingen tot preventie. Onder andere om de mogelijkheid van (aanvullende) preventie nader te onderzoeken is een omvangrijk prospectief onderzoek opgezet.

De opzet is in hoofdstuk 3 beschreven. In de prospectieve studie worden 64 kinderen met hun ouders tijdens en na de opname gevolgd. De patiënten zijn geselecteerd op leeftijd (12 -36 maanden), en de noodzaak van een chirurgische ingreep die naar verwachting tenminste een week ziekenhuisopname impliceert. Ouderparticipatie is het centrale thema. De laatste follow-up is gepland op een zodanige termijn dat volledig herstel van eventuele tijdelijke ontregeling heeft plaatsgevonden: tenminste negen maanden na ontslag. Afhankelijke variabelen hebben betrekking op posthospitalisatie-verschijnselen in de vorm van door de ouders gerapporteerde gedragsproblemen, geobserveerde verstoringen in de interactie tussen het kind en de verzorgende ouder, en testscores voor de receptieve en expressieve taalontwikkeling. Interventies die ten doel hebben de ouderparticipatie te bevorderen werden in een deel van de steekproef op effect beproefd. Elf hypothesen zijn geformuleerd aangaande de determinanten van probleemgedrag na de opname.

Hoofdstuk 4 omvat een beschrijving van de steekproef en de gerealiseerde ouderparticipatie in het ziekenhuis. De experimentele en de controlegroep worden vergeleken in termen van de onafhankelijke variabelen. De medische problemen worden beschreven, het zijn, conform de bedoeling, allerlei verschillende aandoeningen die een indicatie vormen voor chirurgie op deze leeftijd. Voor de helft betreft het afwijkingen die reeds bij de geboorte werden vastgesteld, en vaak heeft al eerder een operatieve ingreep plaatsgevonden. Vervolgens worden de te gebruiken instrumenten psychometrisch doorgelicht en verbeterd. De volgende instrumenten en beoordelingsschalen zijn gereed gemaakt voor de uiteindelijke analyse:

 -opnamegeschiedenis
 -probleemgedrag voorafgaand aan de prospectieve opname
 -sensitiviteit van de ouder (video-opnamen)
 -aanvankelijke gehechtheidskwaliteit (video-opnamen)
 -ouderlijke aanwezigheid/participatie
 -gedragsproblemen op korte en lange termijn
 -verstoring van de relatie met de ouder (video-opname)
 -ego-veerkracht
 -taalontwikkeling relatief tot leeftijd

De toetsing van hypothesen wordt uitgevoerd via covariantie-analyse. De analysemethode en de resultaten zijn in hoofdstuk 6 beschreven. Zowel voorspelde als onverwachte uitkomsten vragen de aandacht. Probleemgedrag is ten dele voorspelbaar uit opnamegeschiedenis, maar op t_1 , d.w.z. voorafgaand aan de prospectieve opname, was dit verband niet, zoals verwacht volgens hypothese (1), statistisch significant. Op t_2 ,twee maanden na ontslag en op t_3 , tenminste negen maanden na ontslag werd de ongunstige invloed van de opnamegeschiedenis manifest in een relatieve toename van probleemgedrag. Uit hypothese (2) kan worden afgeleid dat de zojuist genoemde toename van probleemgedrag zich *niet* zal manifesteren bij (de groep met) een gunstige score voor probleemgedrag in de voortest (t_1). Deze hypothese wordt door de data gesteund.

Hypothese (3) voorspelt dat ouderpaticipatie door interventies zal toenemen. Dit wordt bevestigd. Echter, de gunstige effecten van deze toename op de ontwikkeling van het kind, die werden voorspeld door hypothese (4) blijven geheel uit. Hypothese (5) stelt dat de ontwikkeling na ontslag verband zal houden met de duur van de opname. Dit blijkt, binnen de spreiding van opnameduur die in de steekproef kan worden aangetroffen, niet het geval. In tegenstelling tot hypothese (4) wordt hypothese (6), die inhoudt dat er verband te vinden is tussen ouderlijke ondersteuning gedurende de opname en de latere ontwikkeling wel bevestigd. Dit verband wordt significant bevonden voor de dimensie ouderparticipatie, niet voor de dimensie sensitiviteit. Ouderparticipatie lijkt werkzaam ter voorkoming van verstoringen in de ouder-kind relatie die op t_2 werden geregistreerd en van gedragsproblemen in de laatste follow-up (t_3).

Hypothese (7) heeft betrekking op de verwachting dat veilige gehechtheid een soort bescherming zal bieden tegen ongewenste gevolgen van het ziekenhuisverblijf. Dit wordt niet geconfirmeerd. Veilige gehechte kinderen mét optimale ouderlijke ondersteuning ontwikkelen zich niet ongunstig, maar als de ouderparticipatie te wensen overlaat lijden in deze steekproef juist veilig gehechte kinderen ernstige schade. In hypothese (8) wordt een interactie-effect van opnameduur en ouderparticipatie voorspeld; ook dit wordt niet aangetroffen.

Een belangrijke hypothese die bevestigd wordt is hypothese (9): een gemis aan ouderparticipatie manifesteert zich na het ontslag als vermijdend gedrag tegenover de gehechtheidsfiguur. Vermijdend en negativistisch gedrag werden op t_2 geobserveerd bij de lagere gradatie van ouderparticipatie (die echter nimmer kon worden gekwalificeerd als verwaarlozing). Aan de toetsing van hypothese (10) zijn problemen verbonden die in hoofdstuk 7 aan de orde komen. Hypothese (11) tenslotte, heeft betrekking op de invloed van de ziekenhuisepisode op de taalverwerving. De uitkomsten suggereren het bestaan van een interactie-effect tussen opnamegeschiedenis en (beperkte) ouderparticipatie dat tot een vertraagde spraak/taal ontwikkeling zou kunnen leiden. Bovendien voorspelt verstoring van de relatie, zoals die tot uitdrukking in vermijdend en negativistisch gedrag, een lagere score voor taalbegrip op t_3. Deze beide verbanden hebben te maken met aanwezigheid van de ouders tijdens de opname. De sterkste voorspeller van spraak- en taalontwikkeling bleek echter de sensitiviteit van de ouder.

Uit aanvullende analyses in hoofdstuk 6 blijkt dat rooming-in op zichzelf een rol speelt bij de preventie van verstoringen in de relatie. Het preventief effect geldt voor de steekproef als geheel, maar is het sterkste bij kinderen die een eerste opname hebben doorgemaakt. Voorts wordt in hoofdstuk 6 een vergelijking gemaakt tussen categorieën van aandoeningen wat betreft de psychologische ontwikkeling. Er zijn grote verschillen, die echter gezien moeten worden in het licht van de omvang van de opnamegechiedenis. Het effect op de lange duur wordt uitgedrukt in een effectmaat volgens de formule van Cohen (1977). Het is tamelijk gering in de steekproef als geheel, maar substantieel in de groep met relatief beperkte ouderparticipatie.

Het eerste deel van hoofdstuk 7 omvat een kritische bespreking van de valideit van het prospectief onderzoek. Eén zwakheid is de mogelijkheid dat ouderparticipatie in de controlegroep is versterkt door deelname aan het onderzoek en het beantwoorden van vragen over het kind. Verder worden er aanwijzingen gevonden dat er door antwoordtendenties een systematische vertekening is ontstaan in de rapportage van gedragsproblemen door de ouders kort na ontslag. De externe validiteit van de resultaten is echter goed te noemen.

Onze interpretatie van de uitkomsten houdt in dat *binnen de onderzochte risicogroep* schade aan de kwaliteit van de gehechtheidsrelatie tengevolge van ziekenhuisopname geen zeldzaam verschijnsel is. Vermoedelijk is er een toename van *vermijdende* gehechtheid. Vermijdende gehechtheid is geassocieerd met boosheid jegens de verzorgende ouder. Deze emotionele reactie kan ten dele verklaard worden door de aanvankelijk gepresenteerde theorie; het is echter mogelijk dat de cognitieve onrijpheid van het jonge kind in de beschouwing betrokken moet worden. Het valt te vermoeden dat ouders soms in zekere zin de schuld krijgen van pijn en angst die niet te vermijden zijn. Dit neemt niet weg dat aanwezigheid van de ouder(s) in het ziekenhuis een preventieve waarde heeft.

Aan het slot worden enkele mogelijke richtlijnen voor preventie geformuleerd, op basis van het gerapporteerde onderzoek, in samenhang met de bestaande literatuur:
(a) preventie zou gericht moeten worden op een omschreven leeftijdsfase;
(b) preventie dient gebaseerd te zijn op een conceptie van niet-medisch risico dat ingeschat kan worden door de ziekenhuisstaf;
(c) preventie moet plaatsvinden via de ouders, in de veronderstelling dat ouderparticipatie een beschermende uitwerking heeft;
(d) de autonomie van ouders moet worden gerespecteerd, maar mag niet leiden tot een tekort aan informatie of aanmoediging.

Vier criteria kunnen worden gehanteerd bij de inschatting van het niet-medisch risico:
1. *leeftijd 6 - 36 maanden*
2. *opnameduur: meer dan één of enkele nachten*
3. *opnamegeschiedenis*
4. *symptomen van gebrekkige emotionele aanpassing voorafgaand aan de te verwachten*

ziekenhuisopname

Hier wordt met nadruk bepleit als standaardonderdeel van de planning van een electieve opname een inschatting te maken van het niet-medisch risico en een gesprek aan te gaan over de preventieve waarde van ouderparticipatie. Daarbij kunnen praktische problemen die aanwezigheid van de ouders in het ziekenhuis zouden kunnen belemmeren tijdig aan de orde worden gesteld.

APPENDICES

Appendix 1:   Retrospective questions to parents

Note. The questions are a portion of the original questionnaire selected for relevance to our Chapter 2. They are translated into English to match the rest of the book.

1.1   Parental Questionnaire: attendance in hospital

PQ3   Did you get the opportunity for feeding, washing and clothing your child in hospital?
       (1) no, this was always done by the nurses
       (2) it was mostly done by the nurses; I could help, however
       (3) I could participate every day at fixed hours, at other times this was taken care of by
           the nurses
       (4) the nurses agreed to it that such care was mainly provided by myself
       (5) otherwise: ...

PQ4   Were the children in the ward attended to by a playleader?
       (1) there was no playleader
       (2) there was a playleader, but my child was not much engaged
       (3) my child was regularly attended to by the playleader
       (4) I don't remember

PQ5   What were the regulations for visiting?
       (1) only in the afternoon and the evening
       (2) only in the morning and the afternoon
       (3) in the morning, the afternoon and the evening
       (4) otherwise: ...

PQ6   How often/how much time could you spend to visit your child?
       (1) several times in a week
       (2) about half an hour each day
       (3) about an hour each day
       (4) twice a day, about half an hour
       (5) twice a day, about an hour
       (6) about three hours a day
       (7) three to five hours each day -
       (8) more than five hours each day
       (9) otherwise: ...

PQ7　How often/how much time could your husband spend to visit the child?
(1) several times in a week
(2) about half an hour each day
(3) about an hour each day
(4) twice a day, about half an hour
(5) twice a day, about an hour
(6) about three hours a day
(7) three to five hours each day
(8) more than five hours each day
(9) otherwise: ...

PQ8　Did your child have much pain at the time of hospitalization?
(1) much pain because of the illness or accident
(2) much pain because of medical treatment
(3) much pain by either cause
(4) not so much pain (although hospitalization was distressing)

PQ9　a. Was rooming-in a possibility at the time?
(1) the ward did have provisions for rooming-in
(2) parents could sleep elsewhere in the hospital
(3) there was no possibility for rooming-in
(4) don't know

b. Did you spend the night in the hospital?
(1) no, this could not be managed
(2) yes, I spent ... nights with the child
(3) I spent the night elsewhere in the hospital
(4) rooming-in was unnecessary
(5) otherwise: ...

PQ10　a. Was your child operated upon at this time?
(1) yes
(2) no

b. If yes, were you allowed to be present during
   induction of anaesthesia or during recovery?
(1) neither was allowed
(2) only during induction of anaesthesia
(3) only in the recovery room
(4) present both times
(5) otherwise: ...

Note. The questions have been phrased with a special intent to minimize the influence of social desirability of responses.

120

1.2   Short-term response to hospitalization: 'REA'

REA1 Did your child have trouble either going to bed, or to sleep?
      (1) yes, markedly
      (2) yes, for a while
      (3) no
      (4) I don't remember

REA2 Did your child wake up at night and need comforting?
      (1) frequently; it was a problem
      (2) yes, but not frequently: no severe problem
      (3) no, hardly
      (4) I don't remember

REA3 Was he/she unruly, hard to manage?
      (1) yes, markedly
      (2) yes, for a while
      (3) no
      (4) I don't remember

REA4 Was he/she quick tempered or agressive toward other children or to you?
      (1) yes, frequently
      (2) yes, for a while
      (3) no
      (4) I don't remember

REA5 Did your child present more problems in toilet training?
      (1) he/she did develop such problems
      (2) not markedly
      (3) there were no such problems/toilet training was not yet started
      (4) I don't remember

REA6 Did your child protest being alone in a room?
      (1) yes, markedly
      (2) yes, for a while
      (3) no
      (4) I don't remember

REA7 Did you have the impression that speech development was affected?
      (1) yes, definitely
      (2) maybe
      (3) no
      (4) this is hard to judge

REA8 Was your child wihdrawn after hospitalization?
      (1) yes, markedly
      (2) yes, for a while
      (3) no
      (4) I don't remember

REA9 Did you ever feel the need to consult a professional (social worker, psychologist, pedagogue or therapist)?
(1) not at all
(2) I did not consult anybody, although the need was felt
(3) yes, but this consult was prior to the hospital admission
(4) yes, less than half a year after the hospital admission
(5) yes, but more than half a year after the hospital admission

Appendix 2:   Instructions for scoring disturbance of relationship

Note. The instructions go with Erickson et al. (1985)

2.1   Child's avoidance of mother

This scale reflects the child's tendencies or clear attempts in the session to avoid interacting with the mother. A child high on avoidance would show strong interest *at some point* in the session to withdraw from the mother by leaving the situation or resisting the mother's attempts to engage him or her.
A child low on this scale would show no efforts to avoid the mother *per se*. The child may be angry or noncompliant but yet maintain interaction with the mother.

1.   **Very low**. Child shows no withdrawal from mother. Child maintains roughly an equal level of interaction to mother's interactions throughout the session. If child is noncompliant, some of mother's messages might be ignored, but if it does not seem to be the child's intention to *avoid* interaction with the mother in this situation, such brief ignoring would not count as avoidance.

2.   **Low**. Child shows no clear withdrawal from interaction with mother. Perhaps there is some noncompliance that seems a little suggestive of avoidance and would be counted here.

3.   **Moderately low**. Child has a little tendency to avoid the mother, perhaps through ignoring her for brief periods. There are no major incidents of avoidance, but rather some hints of ambivalence, or lack of interest, about interacting with the mother.

4.   **Moderate**. Child shows some small effort to avoid interaction with mother at some point in the session. There may be a sustained period of ignoring mother's messages or a brief and vague effort to leave the situation. These efforts are easily overcome, however, by moderate pressure by the mother to stay and interact with her.

5.   **Moderately high**. Child makes a clear effort to avoid
interaction with mother. Child's resistance to continued interaction is sustained for some time, but eventually overcome by mother's efforts to maintain the child's involvement with her.

6. **High**. Child has a strongly maintained effort to avoid interaction with mother, probably by repeated attempts to leave the room and avoid contact with her. Once evoked, this avoidance is likely to be repeated unless mother is very cautious in her treatment of child.

7. **Very high**. Child strongly avoids mother for a sustained period and seems highly invested in resisting any emotional bond with her for long periods of the session. Once evoked, the child's avoidance is dominant in the session and remains a possibility to happen again for the rest of the session. Such episodes merit this rating even though the child may have been very engaging of mother earlier in the session.

Note: A child who wants to play with toys in the hallway but does not negotiate this with the mother when she is trying to have him or her stay, and resists mother's efforts to stay, is avoidant. In contrast, a child who wants to leave to play with toys outside, but continues to negotiate with mother about that desire, is *not* avoidant.

2.2 Child's negativity towards mother

Degree to which the child shows anger, dislike, or hostility toward the mother. At the high end, the child is repeatedly and overtly angry at her, e.g., forcefully rejecting her ideas, showing angry and resistant expression, pouting, or being unreasonably demanding or critical of her. At the low end, there are neither overt nor covert signs of such anger. Expressions are essentially positive toward mother whether or not the child is compliant or much involved with her.

1. Child shows no signs of negativism. She/he shows through consistently positive interactions toward the mother that s/he has a truly positive relationship toward her and feels no abiding anger toward her.

2. Child shows no clear indications of negativism, but the tone of some interactions is less positive than one would desire in an ideal relationship toward the mother.

3. Child is negativistic only briefly in any overt fashion, but these suggest some noticeable anger and resistance in the child's interactions with mother.

4. Child shows clear negativism toward the mother on several occasions or one significant occasion, but these are rather isolated episodes separated by periods in which the child behaves quite positively toward the mother.

5. Child is frequently negativistic or shows a few instances of strong or intense negativism, but these are not predominant in the interaction.

6. Child's anger is a predominant aspect of their interactions, but it is shown in more sporadic and generally subtler ways dan in #7.

7. Child is repeatedly and overtly angry or resistant toward the mother. The degree of anger here seems so strong that the child cannot disguise it in subtler ways for long, but it repeatedly appears in her/his interactions with her.

Appendix 3:   Various Statistics

3.1   *ANCOVA concerning effects of time previously spent in hospital with age as covariate*

dependent variables[1]	previous hospital days 0 - 21 n = 44		previous hospital days 22 - 105 n = 20			
	M	(SD)	M	(SD)	F	p^2
t_1 (pretest) BSQ_1	6.3	(4.2)	7.3	(4.7)	.6	.21
t_2 (posttest) BSQ_2	6.2	(3.7)	7.1	(5.4)		
t_3 (long-term) $BSQ_3{}^3$	6.6	(4.5)	8.4	(5.6)		

[1]   high scores on BSQ indicate disadvantage
[2]   p - represents a one-sided probability
[3]   n = 62 at t_3, otherwise n = 64

3.2   *ANCOVAs for effect of previous admissions and parental presence on language development with age and prehospital adjustment as covariates*

	n	comprension quotient N = 62		expression quotient N = 62	
		M	(SD)	M	(SD)
previous admissions 0 or 1					
parental presence 'low'	10	101	(26)	101	(15)
parental presence 'medium/high'	28	93	(20)	95	(21)
previous admissions > 1					
parental presence 'low'	6	76	(11)	75	(11)
parental presence 'medium/high'	18	100	(19)	96	(25)
main effect parental presence		$F (1,57) = .3$		$F (1,57) = 1.4$	
p-value		.59		.23	
main effect previous admissions		$F (1,57) = .0$		$F (1,57) = .7$	
p-value		.93		.39	
parental presence x previous admissions		$F (1,57) = 7.7$		$F (1,57) = 4.2$	
p-value		.01		.04	

3.3 *ANCOVAs for effect of attachment quality and parental presence in hospital on language development with age, previous admissions and prehospital adjustment as covariates*

		comprension quotient $N = 62$		expression quotient $N = 62$	
	n	*M*	*(SD)*	*M*	*(SD)*
secure					
parental presence 'low'	8	86	(18)	84	(20)
parental presence 'medium/high'	27	97	(19)	93	(21)
insecure					
parental presence 'low'	7	97	(32)	100	(15)
parental presence 'medium/high'	15	95	(23)	93	(25)
main effect security		$F (2,53) = .2$		$F (2,53) = 1.5$	
p-value		.86		.23	
main effect parental presence		$F (1,53) = .3$		$F (1,53) = 1.7$	
p-value		.59		.20	
security x parental presence		$F (1,53) = .4$		$F (1,53) = .5$	
p-value		.68		.62	

3.4 *ANCOVAs for effect of attachment quality and disturbed relationship on language development with age, previous admissions and prehospital adjustment as covariates*

		comprension quotient $N = 62$		expression quotient $N = 62$	
	n	*M*	*(SD)*	*M*	*(SD)*
insecure					
disturbed relationship ≤ 3	13	106	(27)	103	(25)
disturbed relationship > 3	9	80	(11)	92	(16)
secure					
disturbed relationship ≤ 3	26	95	(21)	92	(19)
disturbed relationship > 3	9	90	(14)	87	(25)
main effect security		$F (2,53) = .5$		$F (2,53) = 1.6$	
p-value		.63		.21	
main effect dis. relationship		$F (1,53) = 5.1$		$F (1,53) = 2.4$	
p-value		.03		.13	
security x dis. relationship		$F (1,53) = 1.7$		$F (1,53) = .6$	
p-value		.20		.55	

3.5 *Maturation effects of selected BSQ-items, estimated by correlations with age*

BSQ-topic:	correlations with age		
	at t_1	at t_2	at t_3
bedtime resistance	-.16	.05	-.17
sleeping with parents	-.19	.01	-.09
overactivity	.16	.12	.24
attention seeking	.26	.19	-.00
noncompliance	.26	.38	-.00
moodiness	.20	-.12	-.06
total BSQ-score	.15	.01	-.07

REFERENCES

Ainsworth, M.D.S., Blehar, M., Waters, E., & Wall, S. (1978). *Patterns of attachment: A psychological study of the strange situation.* Hillsdale, NJ: Erlbaum.

Ainsworth, M.D.S., & Wittig, B.A. (1969). Attachment and exploratory behavior of one-year-olds in a strange situation. In: B.M. Foss (Ed.), *Determinants of infant behaviour. Vol. 4.* London: Methuen.

Barraclough, W.W. (1937). Mental reactions of normal children to physical illness. *American Journal of Psychiatry, 93,* 865-877.

Bates, J.E., Maslin, C.A., & Frankel, K.A. (1985). Attachment security, mother-child interaction, and temperament as predictors of behavior-problem ratings at age three years. In: I. Bretheton & E. Waters (Eds.), Growing points of attachment theory and theory and research. *Monographs of the Society for Research in Child Development, 50* (1-2, serial no. 209).

Beverly, B.I. (1936). The effect of illness upon emotional development. *Journal of Pediatrics, 8,* 533-543.

Bierman, G. (Ed.) (1978). *Mutter und Kind im Krankenhaus* [Mother and Child in Hospital]. München: Ernst Reinhardt.

Bijstra, J.O., Heyink, J.W., & Tijmstra, Tj. (1991). *Een nieuwe lever, een ander kind? Een onderzoek naar het psycho-sociaal functioneren van kinderen die een levertransplantatie hebben ondergaan* [A new liver, a different child? An inquiry into psychosocial functioning of children after transplantation of the liver]. Groningen: Rijksuniversiteit, Vakgroep Gezondheidswetenschappen.

Block, J.H., & Block, J. (1980). The role of ego-control and ego-resiliency in the organization of behavior. In: W.A. Collins (Ed.), Development of cognition affect and social relations. *Minnesota symposia on Child Psychology,* (13). Hillsdale, NJ: Erlbaum.

Boelen-van der Loo, W.J.C. (1976). *Kinderkliniek* [Pediatric Clinic]. Alphen a/d Rijn: Samsom.

Boer, J.E. de (1992). *De ontwikkeling van de moeder-kind relatie in het eerste levensjaar en de mogelijke invloed van een ziekenhuisopname* [The development of the mother-child relationship during the first year of life and possible impact of hospitalization]. Address to the Association "Kind en Ziekenhuis" at the time of the National Convention, May 1992.

Bowlby, J. (1953). *Child care and the growth of love.* Harmondsworth: Pelican Books.

Bowlby, J. (1969). *Attachment and loss I: Attachment.* London: Hogarth Press.

Bowlby, J. (1969). *Attachment and loss II: Separation, anxiety and anger.* London: Hogarth Press.

Bowlby, J. (1988). The origins of attachment theory. In: J. Bowlby, *A secure base. Clinical applications of attachment theory* (pp. 21-38). London: Routledge.

Brain, D.J., & Maclay, I. (1968). Controlled study of mothers and children in hospital. *British Medical Journal, 1,* 278-280.

Cohen, J. (1988). *Statistical power analysis for the behavioral sciences.* Hillsdale, NJ: Lawrence Erlbaum Associates.

Cook, T.D., & Campbell, D.T. (1979). *Quasi-experimentation: Design and analysis issues for field settings.* Boston: Houghton Mifflin.

Couture, C.J. (1976). The psychological response of young children to brief hospitalization and surgery: the role of the parent-child contact and age. (Doctoral dissertation, Boston University). *Dissertation Abstracts International, 37,* 1427-B.

Damsté, P.H. (1981). *Immuun voor stress: Over weerbaarheid in biologische en sociale zin* [Immune to stress: Concerning resilience in biological and social sense]. Unpublished paper. Utrecht: Rijks Universiteit Utrecht.

Davenport, H.T., & Werry, J.S. (1970). The effect of general anaesthesia, surgery and hospitalization upon the behavior of children. *American Journal of Orthopsychiatry, 40,* 806-824.

Dearden, R. (1970). The psychiatric aspects of the case study sample. In: M. Stacey, R. Dearden, R. Pill, & D. Robinson, *Hospitals, children and their families: Report of a pilot study.* London: Routledge & Kegan Paul.

Douglas, J.W.B. (1975). Early hospital admissions and later disturbances of behaviour and learning. *Developmental Medicine and Child Neurology, 17,* 456-480.

Earls, F., Jacobs, G., Goldfein, D., Silbert, A., Beardslee, W., & Rivinus, T. (1982). Concurrent validation of a behavior problem scale for use with three year olds. *Journal of the American Academy of Child Psychiatry, 21,* 47-57.

Edelston, H. (1943). Separation anxiety in young children. *Genetic Psychological Monographs, 28,* 3-95.

Erickson, M.F., Sroufe, L.A., & Egeland, B. (1985). The relationship between quality of attachment and behavior problems in preschool in a high-risk sample. In: I. Bretherton & E. Waters (Eds.), Growing points of attachment theory and research. *Monographs of the Society for Research in Child Development, 50,* (1-2, serial no. 209).

Fagin, C.M.R.N. (1966). *The effects of maternal attendance during hospitalisation on the posthospital behavior of young children.* Philadelphia: Davis.

Fahrenfort, J.J. (1989). Ziekenhuisopnamen met extra risico [Hospital admissions with extra risk] *Kind en Adolescent, 10,* 1-17.

Fahrenfort, J.J., Jacobs, E.A.M., & Kaptein-de Kock van Leeuwen, M.A.C. (1990). *Prospectief I: Report of a pilot study.* Unpublished report. Leiden: Rijks Universiteit Leiden.

Fahrenfort, J.J., & Kaptein-de Kock van Leeuwen, M.A.C. (1991). Ouderparticipatie bij nuljarigen. [Parental participation in the care of children under one year of age.] *Tijdschrift van de Vereniging Kind en Ziekenhuis, 13,* 104-107.

Faust, J., & Melamed, B.G. (1984). Influence of arousal, previous experience and age on surgery preparation of same day of surgery and inhospital pediatric patients. *Journal of Consulting and Clinical Psychology, 52,* 359-356.

Fischer-Fay, A., Goldberg, S., Simmons, R., Levison, H. (1988). Chronic illness and infant-mother attachment: Cystic fibrosis. *Developmental and Behavioral Pediatrics, 9,* 266-270.

Flavell, J.H. (1979). Metacognition and cognitive monitoring: A new area of cognitive-developmental inquiry. *American Psychologist, 34,* 906-911.

Flavell, J.H., Green, F.L., & Flavell, E.R. (1986). Development of knowledge about the appearance-reality distinction. *Monographs of the Society for Research in Child Development, 51* (1), Serial No. 212.

Forsyth, D. (1934). Psychological effects of bodily illness in children. *Lancet, 227 (I),* 15-18.

Garmezy, N. (1983). Stressors of childhood. In: N. Garmezy & M. Rutter (Eds.), *Stress, coping & development in children.* New York: McGraw Hill.

Goldberger, J. (1987). Supportive environments for infants and toddlers in hospital: What we know, where we are heading, and where we should aim to be. *Children's Environments Quarterly, 4,* 18-24.

Goldsmith, H.H., & Alansky, J.A. (1987). Maternal and infant predictors of attachment: A meta-analytic review. *Journal of Consulting and Clinical Psychology, 55,* 805-816.

Goslin, E.R. (1978). Hospitalization as a life crisis for the preschool child: A critical review. *Journal of Community Health, 3,* 321-346.

Gotowiecz, A., Fischer-Fay, A., & Morris, P. (1990). *Chronic illness, parenting stress and attachment.* Poster presented at the 7th International Conference on Infant Studies Montreal, Quebec.

Hall, D., Pill, R., & Clough, F. (1976). Notes for a conceptual model of hospital experiences as an interactive process. In: M. Stacey (Ed.), The sociology of the national health service. *Sociological Review Monographs, 22.* Keele: University of Keele.

Hall, D., & Stacey, M. (Eds.) (1979). *Beyond separation: Further studies of children in hospital.* London: Routledge and Kegan Paul.

Hannallah, R.S., & Rosales, J.K. (1983). Experience with parents' presence during anaesthesia induction in children. *Canadian Anaesthesiological Society Journal, 30,* 286-289.

Haslum, M.N. (1988). Length of preschool hospitalization, multiple admissions and later educational attainment and behaviour. *Child: Care, health and development, 14,* 275-291.

Hoeksma, J.B., & Koomen, H.M.Y. (1991). *Development of early mother-child interaction and attachment.* (Doctoral Dissertation.) Amsterdam: Vrije Universiteit.

Howells, J.G., & Layng, J. (1955). Separation experiences and mental health: A statistical study. *Lancet, 269 (I),* 285-288.

Hunt, A.D. (1974). On the hospitalization of children: An historical approach. *Pediatrics, 54,* 542-546.

Jackson, K., Winkley, R., Faust, O.A., Cermak, E.G., & Burtt, M.M. (1953). Behavior changes indicating emotional trauma in tonsillectomized children. *Pediatrics, 12,* 23-27.

Jonge, J. de (1985). *Ziekenhuisopname als life-event bij baby's, peuters en kleuters. De lange termijn-effecten daarvan in de vroege adolescentie* [Hospitalization as life-event for infants and prescholars. Long-term effects in early adolescence]. (Postdoctorale scriptie.) Leiden: Rijks Universiteit Leiden.

Kaptein-de Kock van Leeuwen, M.A.C. (1987). *Een onderzoek naar de mogelijke betekenis van pre-operatieve beïnvloeding van ouders en kind voor het psychisch verwerken van het operatietrauma* [An investigation into the efficacy of pre-operative interventions in order to help parents and child in the process of coping with the trauma of surgery.] Master thesis. Leiden: Rijks Universiteit Leiden.

Kaptein-de Kock van Leeuwen, M.A.C., & Jacobs, E.A.M. (1992). *Interventie als preventie?* [Intervention as prevention?] Unpublished report. Leiden: Rijks Universiteit Leiden.

Kind en Ziekenhuis (1982). *Een onderzoek naar enige ziekenhuisvoorzieningen m.b.t. 0-18 jarigen: De situatie in 1982 vergeleken met die van 1977* [An investigation of some provisions in hospitals intended for 0-18 year olds: Situation of 1982 compared to 1977]. Amsterdam: Landelijk Bureau Kind en Ziekenhuis.

Kind en Ziekenhuis (1987). *Een onderzoek naar enige ziekenhuisvoorzieningen m.b.t. 0-18 jarigen: De situatie in 1987 vergeleken met die van 1977 en 1982* [An investigation of some provisions in hospitals intended for 0-18 year olds: Situation of 1987 compared to 1977 and 1982]. Amsterdam: Landelijk Bureau Kind en Ziekenhuis.

Kind en Ziekenhuis (1992). *Welk ziekenhuis kiest u?* [How to choose a hospital]. Dordrecht: Landelijk Bureau Kind en Ziekenhuis.

Knight, R.B., Atkins, A., Eagle, C.J., Evans, N., Finkelstein, J.W., Fukushima, D., Katz, J., & Weiner, H. (1979). Psychological stress, ego defenses and cortisol production in children hospitalized for elective surgery. *Psychosomatic Medicine, 41,* 40-49.

Lambermon, M.W.E. (1991). *Video of folder? Korte en lange termijn effecten van voorlichting over vroegkinderlijke opvoeding* [Video or folder? Short-term and long-term effects of information on early childrearing]. (Doctoral Dissertation.) Leiden: Rijks Universiteit Leiden.

Lehman, E.J. (1975). The effect of rooming-in and anxiety on the behavior of preschool children during hospitalization and follow-up. (Doctoral Dissertation, Cornell University.) *Dissertation Abstracts International, 36,* 3052-B.

Levine, S. (1983). A psychobiological approach to the ontogeny of coping. In: N. Garmezy & M. Rutter (Eds.), *Stress, coping and development in children* (pp. 107-131). New York/ London: McGraw-Hill.

Löschenkohl, E. (1981). Umweltbewältigung bei Kindern in Krankenhaus [Childrens' mastery of the hospital environment]. *Psychologie in Erziehung und Unterricht, 28,* 161-174.

Main, M. (1991). Metacognitive knowledge, metacognitive monitoring, and singular (coherent) vs. multiple (incoherent) models of attachment. In: C.M. Parkes, J. Stevenson-Hinde & P. Harris (Eds.), *Attachment across the life cycle* (pp. 127-159). Tavistock: Routledge.

Mahaffy, P.R. (1965). The effects of hospitalization on children admitted for tonsillectomy or adenoidectomy. *Nursing Research, 14,* 12-19.

McGillicuddy, M.C.A. (1976). A study of the relationship between mothers' rooming-in during their children's hospitalization and changes in selected areas of children's behavior. (Doctoral Dissertation, New York University.) *Dissertation Abstracts International, 37,* 700-B.

Melamed, B.G., Dearborn, M., & Hermecz, D.A. (1983). Necessary considerations for surgery preparation: Age and previous experience. *Psychosomatic Medicine, 45,* 517-525.

Meursing, A.E.E. (1989). Psychological effects of anaesthesia in children. *Current Opinion in Anaesthesiology, 2,* 335-338.

Meyers, E.F., & Muravchick, S. (1977). Anesthesia induction technics in pediatric patients: A controlled study of behavior consequences. *Anesthesia and Analgesia: Current Researches, 56,* 538-541.

Mineka, S., & Suomi, S.J. (1978). Social separation in monkeys. *Psychological Bulletin, 85,* 1376-1400.

Mitchel, G.D., Harlow, H.F., Griffin, G.A, & Möller, G.W. (1967). Repeated maternal separation in the monkey. *Psychonomic Science, 8,* 197-198.

Moore, T. (1969). Stress in normal childhood. *Human Relations, 22,* 235-250.

Mrazek, D.A. (1984). Effects of hospitalization on early child development. In: R.M. Emde & R.J. Harmon (Eds.), *Continuities and discontinuities in development* (pp. 211-225). New York: Plenum Press.

Nagera, H. (1978). Children's reaction to hospitalization and illness. *Child Psychiatry and Human Development, 9,* 3-19.

Olson, S.L., & Bates, J.E. (1978). *Maternal Perception Questionnaire.* Indiana University.

Oremland, E.K., & Oremland, D. (Eds.) (1973). *The effects of hospitalization on children: Models for their care.* Springfield, Illinois: Charles Thomas.

Page, B., & Morgan-Hughes, J.O. (1990). Behaviour of small children before induction: The effect of parental presence and EMLA and premedication with triclofos or a placebo. *Anaesthesia, 45,* 821-825.

Peterson, L. & Shigetomi, C. (1982). One-year follow-up of elective surgery child patients receiving surgery child patients receiving preoperative preparation. *Journal of Pediatric Psychology, 7,* 43-48.

Pinkerton, P. (1981). Preventing psycho-trauma in childhood anaesthesia. In: G.J. Rees & T.C. Gray (Eds.), *Paediatric anaesthesia: Trends in current practice* (pp. 1-18). London: Butterworths.

130

Prugh, D.G., Staub, E.M., Sands, H.H., Kirschbaum, R.M., & Lenihan, E.A. (1953). A study of the emotional reactions of children and families to hospitalization and illness. *American Journal of Orthopsychiatry, 23,* 70-106.

Quinton, D., & Rutter, M. (1976). Early hospital admissions and later disturbances of behaviour: An attempted replication of Douglas' findings. *Developmental Medicine and Child Neurology, 18,* 447-459.

Reynell, J., & Huntley, H. (1977). *Reynell Developmental Language Scales Manual.* Windsor: NFER-Nelson.

Richman, N., & Graham, P.J. (1971). A behavioural screening questionnaire for use with three year old children: Preliminary findings. *Journal of Child Psychology and Psychiatry, 12,* 5-33.

Richman, N., Stevenson, J., & Graham, P.J. (1982). *Preschool to school: A behavioural study.* London: Academic Press.

Riksen-Walraven, J.M.A. (1983). Mogelijke oorzaken en gevolgen van een (on)veilige eerste gehechtheidsrelatie: Een overzicht aan de hand van een model [Possible causes and consequences of (in)secure attachment-relationships: A survey guided by a model]. *Kind en Adolescent, 4,* 23-44.

Robertson, J. (1952). *A two year old goes to hospital.* (16 mm film). Tavistock Child Development Research Unit.

Robertson, J. (1962). *Hospitals and children: A parent's-eye view.* New York: International Universities Press.

Robertson, J. (1970). *Young children in hospital* (second ed. with postscript 1970). London: Tavistock Publications Limited.

Robertson, J., & Robertson, J. (1967). *Young children in brief separation: I. Kate, aged two years five months, in fostercare for 27 days.* Tavistock Child Development Research Unit.

Robertson, J., & Robertson, J. (1968a). *Young children in brief separation: II. Jane, aged 17 months, in fostercare for ten days.* Tavistock Child Development Research Unit.

Robertson, J., & Robertson, J. (1968b). *Young children in brief separation: III. John, aged 17 months, nine days in a residential nursery.* Tavistock Child Development Research Unit.

Robinson, G.C., & Clarke, H.F. (1980). *The hospital care of children: A review of contemporary issues.* Oxford: Oxford University Press.

Roskies, E., Mongeon, D., & Gagnon Lefebvre, B. (1978). Increasing maternal participation in the hospitalization of young children. *Medical Care, 16,* 765-777.

Rutter, M. (1981). *Maternal deprivation reassessed.* Second edition. Harmondsworth: Penguin Books.

Saile, H. (1987). *Psychische Belastung von Kindern durch einen Krankenhaus-aufenthalt: Eine Untersuchung zum Einfluss von Rooming-in und Temperament* [Mental strain of children engendered by hospital admission: An investigation concerning effects of rooming-in and temperament]. Frankfurt am Main: Peter Lang.

Saile, H. (1988). Rooming-in bei Krankenhausaufenthalten von Kindern [Rooming-in during hospital admissions of children]. *Zeitschrift für Klinische Psychologie, 17,* 8-20.

Saile, H., Burgmeier, R., & Schmidt, L.R. (1988). A meta-analysis of studies on psychological preparation of children facing medical procedures. *Psychology and Health, 2,* 107-132.

Schaffer, H.R., & Callender, W.M. (1959). Psychologic effects of hospitalization in infancy. *Pediatrics, 24,* 528-539.

Schofield, N. McC., & White, J.B. (1989). Interrelations among children, parents, premedication and anaesthesists in paediatric day stay surgery. *British Medical Journal, 229,* 1371-1377.

Scholz, C. (1983). *Die Auswirkung der elterlichen Mitaufname (Rooming-in Modell) auf das Verhalten stationär behandelten Kinder: Untersuchung zur poststationären, häuslichen Wiedereingliederung* [The effect of parental rooming-in on the behavior of children after surgery: Investigation of readjustment to home-routines after discharge]. (Doctoral Dissertation.) Berlin: Fachbereich Medizin der Freien Universität Berlin.

Schweizer, A.T. (1978). Mogelijke ontwikkelingen in de psychosociale patiëntenzorg [Developments in psychosocial care of patients]. In: G.M.H. Veeneklaas, A.T. Schweizer, & G.A. Kohnstamm (red.), *Perspectieven in de psychosociale zorg voor het zieke kind* [Perspectives in psychosocial care of diseased infants] (pp 25-27). Deventer: Van Loghum Slaterus.

Simons, B., Bradshaw, J., & Silva, P.A. (1980). Hospital admissions during the first five years of life: A report from the Dunedin multidisciplinary child development study. *New Zealand Medical Journal, 91*, 144-147.

Spencer-Booth, Y., & Hinde, R.A. (1971). Effects of brief separations from mothers during infancy on behaviour of rhesus monkeys 6-24 months later. *Journal of Child Psychology and Psychiatry, 12*, 157-172.

Stacey, M., Dearden, R., Pill, R., & Robinson, D. (1970). *Hospitals, children and their families: Report of a pilot study*. London: Kegan Paul.

Stades Veth, J. (1973). *Spel als signaal: Na ziekenhuisopname van baby of peuter* [Play as symptom: after hospitalization of infant or toddler]. Groningen: Tjeenk Willink. Second edition: Den Haag, Schroeder van der Kolk, 1982.

Stades Veth, J. (1981). *"Verraden door mammie", verstoorde symbiose* ["Betrayed by Mom", disturbed symbiosis]. Den Haag: Vereniging Schroeder van der Kolk.

Stott, D.H. (1956). Effects of separation from the mother in early life. *Lancet, 270 (II)*, 624-628.

Stott, D.H. (1959). Infantile illness and subsequent mental and emotional development. *The Journal of Genetic Psychology, 94*, 233-251.

Swets-Gronert, F. (1986). *Temperament, taalcompetentie en gedragsproblemen van jonge kinderen* [Temperament, language development and behavior problems of young children]. (Doctoral Dissertation, Rijks Universiteit Leiden.) Lisse: Swets en Zeitlinger.

Thompson, R.H. (1985). *Psychosocial research on pediatric hospitalization and health care: A review of the literature*. Springfield: Charles Thomas.

Thompson, R. (1986). Where we stand: Twenty years of research on pediatric hospitalization and health care. *Children's Health Care, 14*, 200-210.

Uitvlugt, M. (1992). *Een hele ingreep* [How to support your child in case of surgery]. Video production for parents. Leiden: Stichting OK&Z.

Van Beek, C.C. (1988). Beleid met creativiteit: Ontwikkelingen in de kinderverpleging [Policy and creativity: Development in pediatric nursing]. *Tijdschrift voor Ziekenverpleging, 42*, 78-84.

Van Bergen, M., & Van Gaalen, M. (1986). *Je kind in het ziekenhuis* [Children in hospital, options for parents]. Utrecht: Kosmos.

Van den Boom, D. (1988). *Neonatal irritability and the development of attachment: Observation and intervention*. (Doctoral dissertation.) Leiden: Rijks Universiteit Leiden.

Van Lieshout, C.F.M., Riksen-Walraven, J.M.A., Ten Brink, P.W.M., Siebenheller, F.A., Mey, J.Th.H. et al. (1986). *Zelfstandigheidsontwikkeling in het basisonderwijs* [Development of independence in primary education]. Nijmegen: Instituut voor Toegepaste Sociologie.

Van IJzendoorn, M.H., & Tavecchio, L.W.C. (1987). Attachment theory as a Lakatosian research program. In: L.W.C. Tavecchio & M.H. van IJzendoorn (Eds.), *Attachment in social networks: Contributions to the Bowlby-Ainsworth attachment theory* (pp. 3-26). Amsterdam: North-Holland Publishing Company.

Van IJzendoorn, M.H., & Kroonenberg, P.M. (1988). Crosscultural patterns of attachment: A meta-analysis of the Strange Situation. *Child Development, 60,* 728-737.

Van IJzendoorn, M.H., Goldberg, S., Kroonenberg, P.M., & Frenkel, O.J. (1992). The relative effects of maternal and child problems on the quality of attachment: A meta-analysis of attachment in clinical samples. *Child Development, 63,* 840-858.

Veeneklaas, G.M.H., Gobée, J., & Van der Kloot-Meijburg, W. (1972). *Kind en ziekenhuis: De derde persoon aan het ziekbed* [Child & hospital: The third person at the bedside]. Leiden: Stenfert Kroese.

Vernon, D.T.A., & Schulman, J.L. (1964). Hospitalization as a source of psychological benefit to children. *Pediatrics, 34,* 694-696.

Vernon, D.T.A., Foley, J.M., Sipowicz, R., & Schulman, J.L. (1965). *The psychological responses of children to hospitalization and illness.* Springfield: Thomas.

Vernon, D.T.A., Schulman, J.L., & Foley, J.M. (1966). Changes in children's behavior after hospitalization: Some dimensions of response and their correlates. *American Journal of Diseases of Children, 111,* 581-593.

Vernon, D.T.A., & Bailey, W.C. (1974). The use of motion pictures in the psychological preparation of children for induction of anaesthesia. *Anaesthesiology, 40,* 68-72.

Wanschura, T., & Löschenkohl, E. (1979). Kind im Krankenhaus: Zwei Bedingungsmodelle für die Verstärkung/Hemmung von Verhaltensstörungen [Child in hospital: Two models of the factors that increase or reduce behavioral disturbance]. *Praxis der Kinderpsychologie und Kinderpsychiatrie, 28,* 51-55.

Waters, E., Wippman, J., & Sroufe, L.A. (1979). Attachment, positive affect and competence in the peer group: Two studies in construct validation. *Child Development, 50,* 821-829.

Wolfer, J.A., & Visintainer, M.A. (1979). Prehospital psychological preparation for tonsillectomy patients: Effects on children's and parent's adjustment. *Pediatrics, 64,* 646-655.

Woodward, J. (1959). Emotional disturbances of burned children. *British Medical Journal, 1,* 1009-1013.

Woodward, J.M. (1962). Parental visiting of children with burns. *British Medical Journal, 2,* 1656-1657.

Yap, J.N. (1988a). The effects of hospitalization and surgery on children: A critical review. *Journal of Applied Developmental Psychology, 9,* 349-358.

Yap, J.N. (1988b). A critical review of pediatric preoperative preparation procedures: Processes, outcomes and future directions. *Journal of Applied Developmental Psychology, 9,* 359-389.

ACKNOWLEDGEMENTS / DANKBETUIGINGEN

Aan de randvoorwaarden voor uitvoering van het gerapporteerde onderzoek kon worden voldaan dankzij de subsidie van het Praeventiefonds en de plaats die hiervoor binnen de Vakgroep Algemene Pedagogiek werd ingeruimd. Ideeën van Prof. Dr P.H. Damsté hebben de kiem gelegd voor de theorie, die verder is ontwikkeld met behulp van experts die deel uitmaken van de promotiecommissie. Voor adviezen van wetenschappelijke aard komt tevens dank toe aan Prof. Dr Ph. Treffers en aan Dr Dymph van den Boom, die ook hielp bij het beoordelen van gehechtheidskwaliteit. Daarnaast heeft het project in een vroeg stadium de steun ondervonden van Drs Sjoeke van der Meulen, Dr F.A. Swets-Gronert, kinderpsychiater J. de Jonge en mevrouw C.C. van Beek.

Een belangrijk aandeel in de uitvoering van het onderzoek hadden Drs Gidia Jacobs en Drs Marguérite Kaptein-de Kock van Leeuwen. Adviesgesprekken met ouders van kinderen die op de nominatie stonden voor ziekenhuisopname werden door Marguérite gevoerd. Aan het verzamelen van de gegevens werd ook door Corrie van Staalduinen een belangrijke bijgedrage geleverd. Beoordelingen van video-materiaal werden volgens strikte instructies uitgevoerd door Drs Gidia Jacobs, Drs Juchke van Roozendaal (sensitivity) en Drs Arja de Jong (disturbed relationship). Drs C. Schuengel assisteerde bij het retrospectief onderzoek. Het secretariaatswerk voor het jarenlange onderzoekproject werd steeds verricht door Carla Hermsen. Bart Bosman hielp bij het persklaar maken van het proefschrift.

De heren A. van der Zaan, J.W.M. van der Velde en L. Star van de audiovisuele dienst hielpen geweldig door alle technische apparatuur te verzorgen en video-materiaal te dupliceren. Mevrouw I. Weber zorgde voor het opvragen van veel materiaal ten behoeve van de literatuurstudie.

Veel dank komt toe aan de ziekenhuismedewerkers, die zich soms een extra taak op de hals haalden door hun onmisbare medewerking aan het signaleren en werven van respondenten: Mary Gadella en Corry Los van het Juliana Kinderziekenhuis, Nel van Deutekom, Karin Vink en Dr J. Ottenkamp van het Academisch Ziekenhuis Leiden, Carolina van Soest, Dr J.M. Nijman en Dr F.W.J. Hazebroek van het Sophia Kinderziekenhuis, Ielka Eisinga van het AZVU, Ellie van Vliet, Lenie Paap en Drs A.L.T. van Overbeek-van Gils van het Reinier de Graafziekenhuis, Sandra Roodbergen en Drs R. Rodrigues-Pereira van het St Clara-Ziekenhuis. Aan het retrospectief onderzoek werd meegewerkt door mevrouw G.C. de Vrij van het AZL, de heer J. Steffin van het Diaconessenhuis te Leiden en de heer J.P. Kloos van het Merwedeziekenhuis in Dordrecht.

De belangrijkste plaats waar het erkentelijkheid betreft komt toe aan de ouders die als respondenten aan het onderzoek hebben deelgenomen. Hun bereidwilligheid om ondanks eigen problemen een bijdrage te leveren was vaak hartverwarmend en vanzelfsprekend onmisbaar.

CURRICULUM VITAE

Joop Fahrenfort was born in Amsterdam in 1944. He attended gymnasium (B) in Den Helder. He studied initially mathematics and philosophy, later psychology at the University of Amsterdam. He obtained his first degree (*doctoraal*) in psychology c.l. in 1972, specializing in methodology of research. Subsequently he taught statistics at Brabant University (KUB), participated in research on foster children at Leiden University (RUL), conducted research on psychomotor therapy in Amsterdam (VU), and research on prevention of atopic allergy in Utrecht (RUU). He did other things besides. The project concerning *Attachment and Early Hospitalization* was hatched and nurtured in Leiden.